Living the WELLNESS Lifestyle

Transform Your Life: Look Younger, Feel Better, Live Healthier!

Originally published as
The Wellness Lifestyle!: Look Great, Feel Great,
and Defy the Signs of Aging!

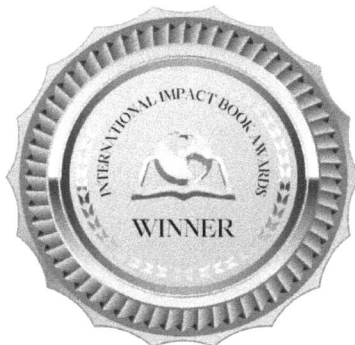

INTERNATIONAL IMPACT BOOK AWARDS
WINNER

ii

See what people are saying about Dr. Wanda on Google Reviews

Joyce said...

★★★★★

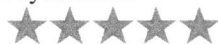

After experiencing symptoms that I suspected were related to some of the foods that I was eating, I started seeing Holistic Health Functional Wellness. During our first appointment, she asked me every possible question so she could get a full picture of my health, from the specifics of what I eat, to how much I sleep, to my activity levels, everything. I completed an MRT Food Sensitivity test, which was very detail-oriented and lengthy. I was very happy to see that some of my questions were finally answered. The results were outstanding because some of the healthy food, I was eating was causing my problems such as pineapple, garlic, coconut, and turkey. She went over my Mediator Release Test (MRT) results and explained my reaction level (Low, Moderate, and High) and I followed a restricted food plan for a month where I was only allowed to eat certain foods, and I gradually added additional foods. After a week following these restrictions, I immediately noticed that my stomach was no longer bloated, and I started losing 2 pounds a week, and sleeping 7 hours a night. She welcomes emails with questions, concerns, and we met online live every 2 weeks to discuss any concerns, test results, etc. Bottom line: I highly recommend that anyone with health concerns consult her.

Judie said...

★★★★★

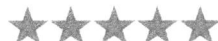

Working with Wanda has been a wonderful experience one that I have been search-ing for a long time. I have finished the program and will continue to follow what I have learned about my body. Wanda is a great listener and has a holistic approach to treat inflammation that is easy to understand and follow. Invest in yourself with Wanda.

Nicky said...

★★★★★

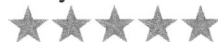

It was great learning healthy habits with Dr. Wanda. She gave us the needed tools to succeed in forming new and healthy habits. She also did a hair analysis helping me to identify my mineral deficiencies and provide me the needed resources to improve my health. I am a health professional myself, but I was not educated on functional medicine. However, this is the way our society needs to work toward. Healthcare has become a business model of greed. The providers are not well-versed in prevention.

More Google Reviews

Sherrie said...
★★★★★

In my wellness journey, I've attempted to learn about holistic ways to solve some of my health problems but it wasn't until I started working with Dr. Wanda Parks that I started seeing results. Her teaching, guidance, and accountability were key...to my understanding and steadfastness in staying on track. My one-on-one meetings were exceptional. Taking the time to listen and follow her instructions, also caused my hubby and kids to become curious and they joined in on the wellness journey.
With Dr. Parks' assistance, my family learned from me as I learned from her, so we began eating healthier, exercising together, journaling wellness habits, and had fun while doing so. Let her teach you how to lead your family into a healthy lifestyle change.

Angela said...
★★★★★

Dr. Wanda is very knowledgeable and passionate about holistic health. I'm so glad I found her! I look forward to a long-lasting holistic health relationship.

Yolanda said...
★★★★

The program was very detailed and informative.

BOOKS BY DR. WANDA PARKS

The Wellness Lifestyle!: Look Great, Feel Great, and Defy the Signs of Aging! 1st Edition

30-Day Living Your Created Life Reflective Food Journal: Manifesting Your Dream one Day at a Time

Books Co-authored by Dr. Wanda Parks

You Were Made To Be Unstoppable: A Collection of Unstoppable Stories That Will Inspire You to Believe Bigger

SECOND EDITION

Living the
WELLNESS
Lifestyle

Transform Your Life:
Look Younger,
Feel Better,
Live Healthier!

DR. WANDA PARKS
I-MD, PHD, MA, BSN, FDN-P

DAYNA OFFUTT
digital designs

PUBLISHING

Living Your Created Life, LLC DBA
Holistic Health Functional Wellness

www.successwithwanda.com
wanda@successwithwanda.com

ISBN: 979-8-9923560-0-7

Parks, Dr. Wanda.
Living the Wellness Lifestyle - Transform Your Life: Look Younger, Feel Better, Live Healthier!

Cover design: Dayna Offutt
Formatting and design layout: Dayna Offutt
Photography: Christen Parks Photography
Images: The images used for this project are from Ideogram.ai, Creative Fabrica, and Unsplash.

CONTENTS

FOREWORD

Take charge of your personal wellness, empower yourself with knowledge, approach life (and the challenges of life) with positivity, develop a 'can do' mindset —all strong messages that come through with vision and clarity in Wanda's book, *Living the Wellness Lifestyle - Transform Your Life: Look Younger, Feel Better, Live Healthier!*

Having known Wanda professionally for several years, we developed a friendship that led me to realize her passion for educating and inspiring others to achieve improved overall wellness. This passion came, in part, from her own lived life experience and challenges, and her perspective as a nurse. This experience grounds her in how she views the journey of wellness as being very unique and individualized. She appreciates that each individual has strengths and challenges that can change from year to year or even day to day.

In this easy-to-read book, Wanda inspires readers to explore six key areas that can contribute to overall wellness. She provides inspiration and information in all key areas and ultimately provides action steps to help break it all down into bite-sized pieces. This approach helps guide readers to strategies that can positively impact their overall personal wellness. Her positive, 'can do' message can help readers move forward to achieve their wellness goals and live the life they love.

Dr. Julie Baldwin
DNP, RN

PREFACE

Well hello, and thank you for getting this book.

I have poured my heart and soul into it, and I hope that the information contained within helps you to get everything you want when it comes to feeling amazing and having the life you deserve.

Let's dive right in, because I have a quick question for you...

Let's say you are out to lunch and you see two women enjoying lunch together. One is slender and wears size six clothing, and the other is twenty pounds overweight.

Who is healthier?

Wait a moment before you answer, because this is a trick question. The fact is, we do not know enough to say who is healthier from just this basic information. Maybe that is not earth-shattering news, but there was a time when it was a revelation to me.

Now I am going to ask you what may sound like a really basic question, but here's the thing—I want you to really think about this.

Mull it over, let it sink in and come up with your own answer. There is no right or wrong to this, but to get you started in the right direction, I really need you to do this exercise.

Are you ready?

There are actually two questions...

What does being healthy and well mean to YOU?

Seriously—how do you know that you are truly well, that you are healthy, and that you are physically, emotionally and mentally fit?

When I finally sat down and asked myself these questions, I realized that I didn't have a clue.

However, I can tell you this—when I personally embarked on my own wellness journey, this reflection was a critical first step. I initially focused on weight as the ultimate marker of wellness. The lower the weight (within reason) the better, right?

You may already know this wasn't very smart on my part.

Obviously, there is much more to wellness than just a reading on a scale. As I was continuing to explore 'wellness,' I had began to realize how multi-dimensional this seemingly simple word really is.

As a nurse, I understand the scientific functioning of the various body systems. This basic functioning is critical; however, I felt there was much more. In order to really experience true wellness in my own life, I needed to address these six areas, or you may call them spectrums. See Figure 1-1.

Dr. Wanda's *SPECTRUM OF WELLNESS*

Mental	Physical	Social	Environmental	Spiritual	Financial

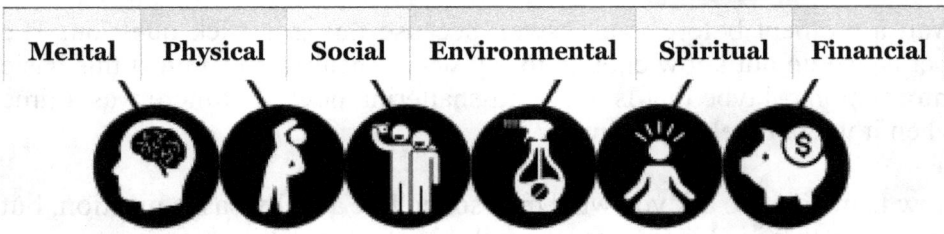

Figure 1-1: Dr. Wanda's *6 Spectrums of Wellness* are essential to gain the benefits of living the wellness lifestyle!

Until I had cultivated *every single one* of these areas, I knew I would not be able to experience a total wellness that would allow my life to go from good to fantastic!

I had a friend who purchased a 100-year-old farmhouse. The thing was, the house was sagging on one corner. I mean the house was actually shifting and sinking! If something was not done soon, the house would be beyond repair and would have to be torn down. My friend hired an expert to fix the house. What he did was literally jack up the sinking corner of the house as if you might jack up a car, and then put in permanent jacks to shore it up. Crazy, right? However, it worked like a charm. The house was level, it was beautifully done, it looked like new, and you would never know there had ever been anything wrong with it. At a certain point in my wellness journey, I realized I was looking at wellness like the foundation of a house.

If the foundation begins to shift in even just one area, it can severely impact the integrity of the entire structure. Walls crack, pipes break, windows burst, support beams bend, ceilings fall, the entire weight shifts and soon it is beyond repair.

As I assessed my own personal foundation, I realized there were a few cracks and areas I could strengthen. As I began to work on these areas, I realized every aspect of my life felt more in sync, more stable, and more solid.

I was beginning to experience that overall feeling of wellness. As time progressed and I did more work, my foundation became more solid. Finally, I could experience wellness in a way that was completely transforming, uplifting and life affirming!

Somewhere along this journey, I realized my calling was to help others achieve this amazing feeling of wellness. That is why I am so happy you have decided to let me be your guide toward total wellness. I realize this journey is very individualized, but taking time to assess your own personal foundation and then taking steps to fix those annoying cracks in the foundation can be truly life transforming. So, let's get started!

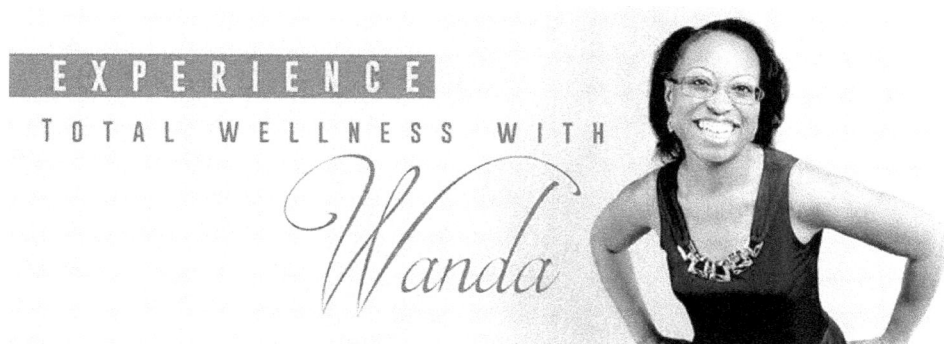

EXPERIENCE
TOTAL WELLNESS WITH
Wanda

ACKNOWLEDGEMENTS

First, I would like to acknowledge God, who is the head of my life and my strength. Who has given me a vision and the ability to see it through.

My husband, David Parks, who is my Chief Supporting Officer (CSO). He has supported and stood by me through all my endeavors. His unselfish love has kept me motivated and inspired.

My children, Kevin, DJ, and Kaneshia who I love dearly. They, too, have always supported me through all of my educational journeys, and business endeavors as well as during the hectic times when I was 'very busy,'—they understood and continued to display their unwavering love to see us all through.

My 'Sister'—Cousin, Rhonda, whom I can depend on to vent to, and who is able to encourage me when I feel a bit discouraged. She is always in my corner.

Finally, Dr. Julie Baldwin, DNP, RN, who was the inspiration for me even starting my journey in sharing my passion and helping formulate my vision to educate and mentor others on true wellness.

Meet Dr. Wanda

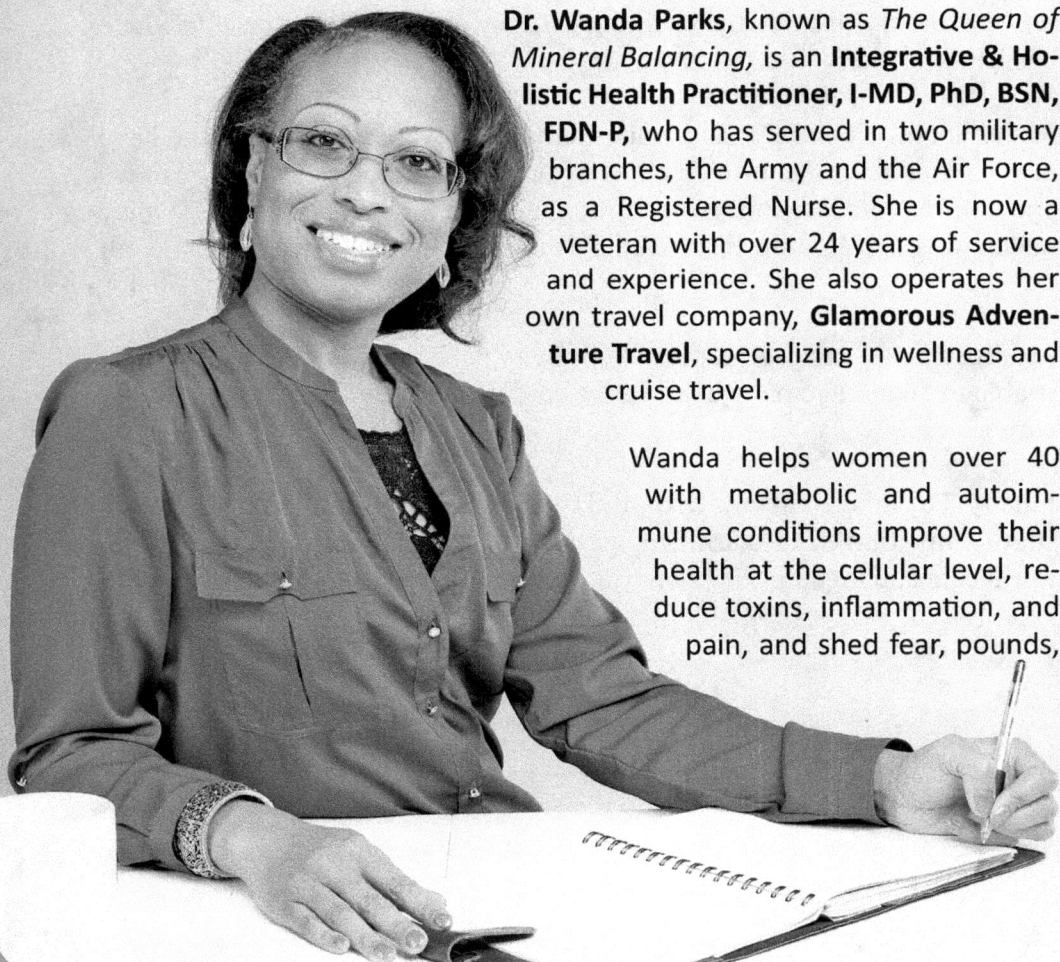

Dr. Wanda Parks, known as *The Queen of Mineral Balancing,* is an **Integrative & Holistic Health Practitioner, I-MD, PhD, BSN, FDN-P,** who has served in two military branches, the Army and the Air Force, as a Registered Nurse. She is now a veteran with over 24 years of service and experience. She also operates her own travel company, **Glamorous Adventure Travel**, specializing in wellness and cruise travel.

Wanda helps women over 40 with metabolic and autoimmune conditions improve their health at the cellular level, reduce toxins, inflammation, and pain, and shed fear, pounds,

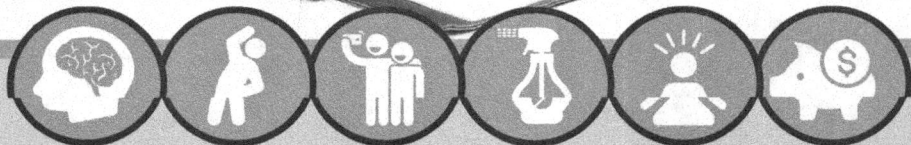

The Queen of
Mineral Balancing

and self-doubt. She treats every cell, tissue, organ, and system in the body simultaneously, looking for health revitalization opportunities.

Wanda is a certified Aromatherapist, Face Yoga Instructor, and Flexibility Yoga Coach. She is a two-time published author of *The Wellness Lifestyle* and *The 30-Day Living Your Created Life: Reflective Food Journal,* and a #1 Best-Selling Co-Author of *You Were Made to be Unstoppable.* Wanda offers a unique approach to wellness, including several programs; her core offering is her *90-day Body Awareness Gut Detox Program.* She also offers the *Total Body Transformation System*, her premier 7-month program, which includes seven functional lab screenings particularly unique, focusing on identifying opportunities to improve wellness.

If you are new to holistic health, Dr. Wanda offers *'The Holistican' Wellness Membership.* She believes functional wellness is paramount to improving your wellbeing. She teaches people how to take control of their health and wellness naturally, without relying on yo-yo and fad diets, enabling them to live a more energetic, vibrant lifestyle.

Wanda has earned dual Bachelor's degrees in Nursing and Holistic Health, and dual Master's degrees in Human Resource Management and Military Operational Arts. Additionally, she holds a PhD and a Doctorate in Integrative Medicine.

❧ Living the ❧
WELLNESS
Lifestyle

Transform Your Life:
Look Younger,
Feel Better,
Live Healthier!

INTRODUCTION

Now before we get into the six spectrums of wellness, I would like to speak to you about your mindset.

I know, I know – you want to get into the 'meat' of the book. Mindset isn't important, right? You know you need to think positive and now let's just move on.

I understand that mindset. However, here's what I need to convey to you – the biggest, boldest, most effective thing you can do to improve your physical health and well-being is to improve your mindset.

If you are not in the right place mentally, then nothing I teach you here is going to be of much value to you.

You must be ready for what you are about to discover. You have to realize there's no magic fix, and everything we talk about here will take work. (Yes, I know work is a 4-letter word, but it is a GOOD 4 letter word once you realize it is the surest way to success.)

Paradoxically, everything I teach you here will be easy, but it will also take work. Therefore, I want you to think about why you chose this book, what you want to change in your life and why you're ready to change it. There are six spectrums we will be going through, and we are going to help you in each area.

You may not adapt to all of these changes 100%, but there are some things you can change in each of the six spectrums, to guide you to achieve total wellness or balance in your life. Nevertheless, your mindset should be ready first. In addition, you must be determined to succeed.

Here are some foundational questions for you—please answer them to your own satisfaction. After all, the more you put into this process, the more you will get out of it.

What is your *'why?'*

Why do you want to look younger and feel better?

Why do you want to live healthier? Moreover, why do you want to have more energy? Who is this going to help? What is the main goal behind your gaining an understanding of the total spectrum of wellness?

As we already discussed, this is not just about weight loss.

I would like you to delve in and get the big picture of your overall wellness goals and what you would like to discover in each of these chapters.

Remember to take the Action Steps at the end of each chapter, and do not rush through this book. This will guide you and allow you to obtain the results you seek.

"When we fill our
thoughts with
the right things,
the wrong ones
have no room to enter"

~ Joyce Meyer

1

MENTAL WELLNESS

Have you ever thought: 'I'm not good enough, I'll never be anything, I'll never amount to anything,' 'Why do bad things always happen to me,' or 'How come I'm not lucky like that person?'

Conversely, have you ever thought, 'I'm the greatest, I'm amazing, I could do anything and I'm successful?'

These types of thoughts are part of your mental wellness. If your thoughts are negative, that is what you are going to attract in your wellness life.

You are going to attract stress and a lot of negativity. This is because you are always attracting what you are constantly thinking and speaking about. However, if your thoughts are positive, you are going to attract positive people, great opportunities, and success.

Mental wellness pertains to your mindset and your thoughts. It is maximizing positive emotions and being able to cope in a stressful situation, whether that stressful situation is good or bad. An example would be the death of a loved one. Obviously, that is a bad incident and can cause negative stress. Getting married is an example of positive stress. Divorce, of course, depends on how you look at it – it might be happy or sad, good or bad stress. The same goes for the birth of a child.

Changes in your life are continually putting positive and negative stresses into your life and affecting your mental wellness. Your mental wellness is not just important, it is crucial. If your mindset is not right, then you cannot cope through stressful situations. It makes sense, right? When you have negative thought processes, negative thinking, or you are always saying negative things, then you may become more depressed and you do not cope as well. In addition, this inevitably leads to destructive behavior.

According to a Harris poll done in 2013, only 33% of people consider themselves happy. I was initially shocked when I read this, but now I realize it's likely true. If you look at yourself and your two best friends, odds are, only one of you considers yourselves happy most of the time.

Happiness is part of your mental wellness and many different things have the potential to make you feel happy. It is important to note here that mental wellness and physical wellness work hand-in-hand with the amount and type of exercise you get. When you exercise, you release endorphins, which make you happy. These endorphins create a better mood for you, and when you are in this better mood, others want to be around you, too.

Your mental wellness can also be affected by your nutrition. What you eat affects how you feel, not just physically but also mentally. For example, healthy fats can help with Alzheimer's, improve your concentration, and enhance your ability to remember things.

Are you beginning to see why mental wellness is crucial to achieving total wellness?

When you are not mentally well, this can lead to depression, which can also affect your physical wellness. This is why your mental health and wellness is important to achieving your total wellness.

When you have great mental wellness, your coping skills are better. Having a great support system of family or friends will also help you to cope through any changes in your life. In addition, if you also have positive thinking as a coping mechanism, you are more likely to find and/or create circumstances that lead to overall happiness.

Having a healthy mental wellness that gets you up in the morning and gets you going, will help you to achieve your goals. You will be able to brush off the smaller negative things in life that hit you. After all, we are all going to go through some negativity and some challenges in life, and the time to prepare for those events is before they happen.

One of the things that helps with your mental well-being is eating a healthy diet. Your brain is part of your mental wellness and you need to have a great functioning brain, which of course runs on food. You can see how all of these things are closely interconnected. You need to be aware of what fuels your brain to help you with your thought processes and your memory.

You want to protect your mental health so you can have a productive life. If you want to enjoy your grandchildren and some of you may want to enjoy your great-grandkids—then you really want to make sure you nourish your mental wellness.

This way you can have that vibrant memory recalling some wonderful things in your life, you will be more readily able to tune out the negative experiences, learn valuable lessons from them, and begin having a refreshing life as you age.

If there are negative thoughts that pop into your mind, you will want to replace those thoughts with positive ones. Why do you need to do that? Because it will help you to get more clarity, to focus on your goals, and help propel you to where you want to go.

Another way to aid in your mental wellness is meditation: Meditation is a mind and body practice. There are many types of meditation, most of which originated in ancient religious and spiritual traditions. Some forms of meditation instruct the practitioner to become mindful of thoughts, feelings, and sensations and to observe them in a nonjudgmental way.

Many studies have investigated meditation for different conditions, and there is evidence that it may reduce blood pressure as well as symptoms of irritable bowel syndrome and flare-ups in people who have had ulcerative colitis. It may ease symptoms of anxiety and depression and may help people with insomnia.

Meditation may also help with the following:

Pain	*Smoking Cessation*
Insomnia	*Other Conditions*

Here is a quick meditation you can try right now:

Get comfortable in a quiet place. Become present in the moment.

When your mind wanders (and it will) just bring it back to the present. It might help to focus on a tiny dot of light in your mind.

Pay close attention to your breathing. Take slow breaths in, and slow breaths out.

Feel your body. Notice each sensation.

Practice. You might get frustrated at first, and that is okay. Just keep practicing and you will get better and better at it.

MENTAL ACTION TASKS

Do you have a support system?

☐ Yes　　　☐ No

If so, list them here. If not, list the names of those you would like to be a part of your support system.

1		7	
2		8	
3		9	
4		10	
5		11	
6		12	

If you do not already have a dozen friends you can call at the drop of a hat, I suggest you get to work finding and making these friends. *The time to make new friends is always before you need them!*

How often do you complain each day?

☐ Rarely　　　☐ Quite often　　　☐ Constantly

Keep a running tally—you might be surprised! When you find yourself complaining, silently remind yourself that you no longer wish to continue in that behavior pattern, and choose instead to look at the positive side of the situation.

Are the bulk of your thoughts positive or negative?

☐ Mostly negative　　　☐ Both negative & positive　　　☐ Mostly positive

Each time you have a negative thought, correct yourself and turn it into a positive thought. Over time, you will find that positive thinking becomes more natural to you.

Do you see the glass as half full or half empty?

☐ Half full　　　☐ Half empty

Being optimistic does not mean being a Pollyanna. Rather, it is a philosophy of always looking for and finding the good in situations, and expecting positive rather than negative outcomes.

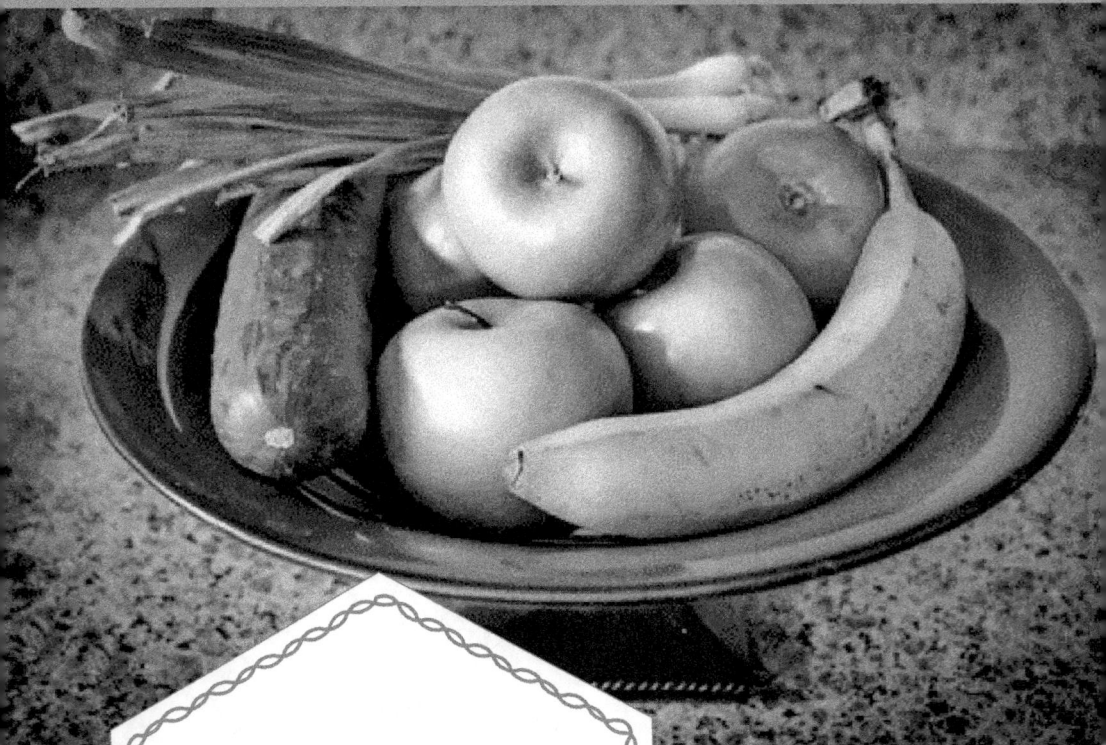

"Eating well is
a form of
respecting your
temple"

Image Credit:
Christen Parks Photography

PHYSICAL WELLNESS

Have you ever felt like the activities you once loved doing are now beyond your reach? Maybe you are feeling stagnant and stiff, or you have no energy and you have gained a few extra pounds.

Let's face facts—the body you used to have is not the same body you have today. Believe me; I know exactly how that feels!

Worse yet, you cannot seem to get your old body back. What is the problem? You don't know, but it sure is frustrating, isn't it? Here is what is happening in a nutshell:

Your physical wellness is being attacked. Physical wellness has been defined as *promoting proper care of our bodies for optimal health and functioning.*

In addition, just like overall wellness, physical wellness can be multidimensional. Physical wellness is a critical piece of our overall wellness foundation.

As I explored the dimensions of physical wellness, I came up with four main categories: Nutrition, Exercise, Sleep/rest, and Stress Reduction. These four are major foundational blocks for our physical wellness to function. So let's take a little closer look at each one of these.

#1 NUTRITION

Nutrition provides us with the fuel we need to engage in the game of life.

Without proper nutrition, your body is unable to run smoothly and efficiently. Try to think of your body as an automobile. Would you rather be a smooth running sports car or a sputtering clunker?

Nutrition plays a major role in how our engine runs. Nutrients are what our bodies need for growth, maintenance and repair. Water is one of the main nutrients—like oil is to the car engine.

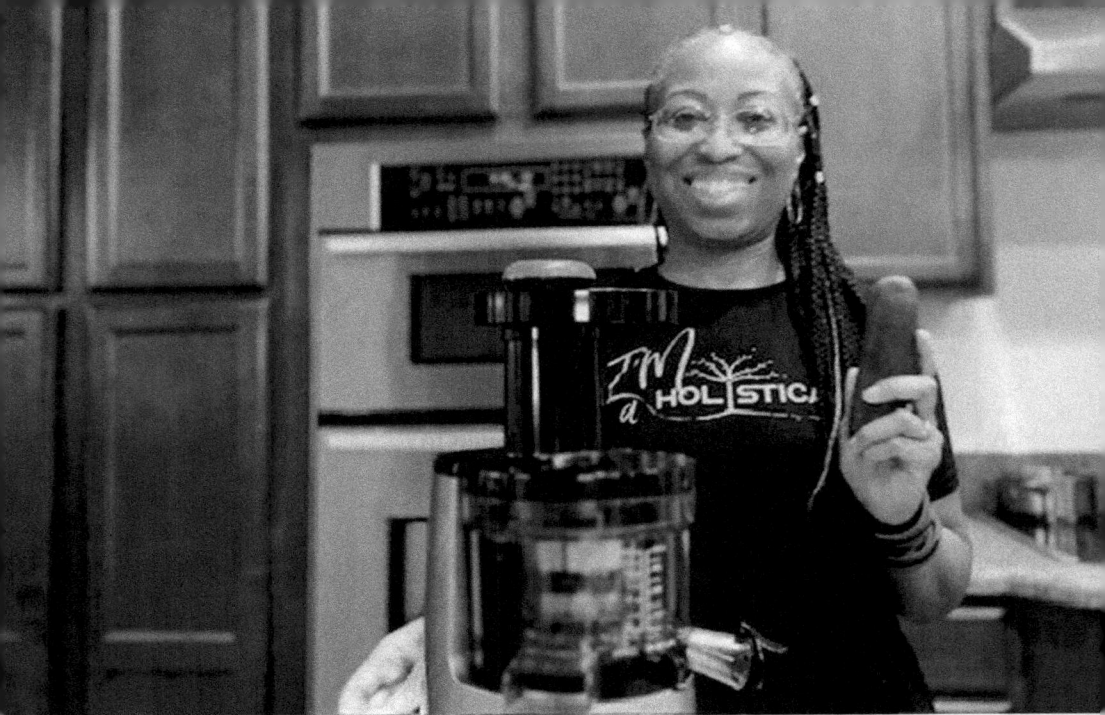

There are five additional categories of nutrients to consider: Carbohydrates, protein, fats, vitamins, and minerals.

Grab my free report from the link below, to get more in-depth with these nutrients at: ***https://solo.to/drwanda***

Do you know what my #1 tip is for getting the nutrition you need? Smoothies! Choose green or red. Invest in a high-end blender such as a Vitamix, or any pulverizing blender.

Green Smoothie*
1   *Purchase fresh greens such as kale, chard, spinach, and cucumber.*
2   *Mix greens with fresh fruits, milk, yogurt, and anything healthy you choose.*
3   *Throw in a banana and a carrot or two, and enjoy!*
* If you prefer to go for the Red Smoothie, purchase items such as raspberries, blackberries, and strawberries and mix with some almond milk, vanilla, and other healthy choices. You can also throw a bit of green in your red, and enjoy!

A pulverizing blender will pulverize everything into a rich, creamy drink you can enjoy daily. The nutrients in all the greens and reds will be easily digested by your body—no chewing required!

#2 EXERCISE

Exercise is the second component in physical wellness. Our bodies are built to move. Movement is vital to prevent you from becoming stiff. I once heard someone say, *'motion is lotion,'* meaning that movement helps to keep our joints more supple and ready for movement. Similar to the way that oil lubricates the engine pistons.

Exercise also helps strengthen your muscles and increases muscle mass. *With more muscle mass, you are able to stay in a fat-burning mode longer, which can aid in weight management.* Exercise releases endorphins, those 'feel good' hormones. Exercise can increase your energy, helps with aging, improves memory, increases happiness and helps you to sleep better.

Some doctors are now promoting *'Exercise is Medicine.'* Exercise has slowly developed through recent global dissemination. Exercise is one of the top modifiable risk factors for chronic disease. *This means by increasing your exercise – both how much you exercise and how often – you can reduce your risk of most chronic diseases.*

To stay active, you only need to walk for 30 minutes a day or 45 minutes, three times a week. Just be sure to consult with your physician before starting any exercise program.

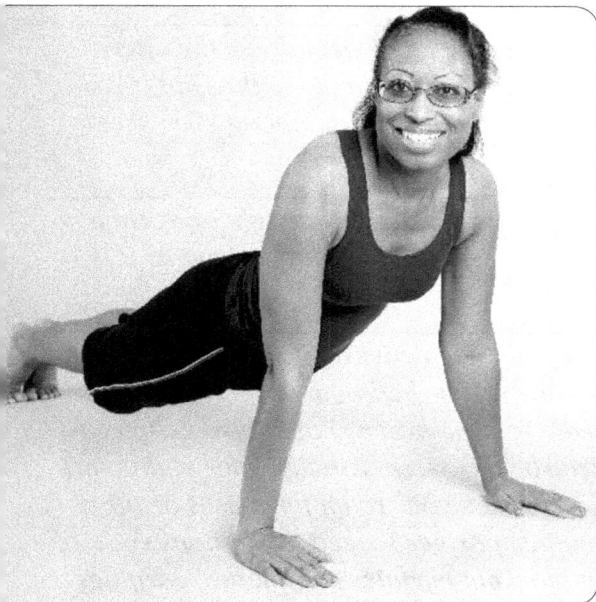

#3 SLEEP AND REST

Sleep and rest is the third component of physical wellness. There is a difference between *sleep* and *rest*. Sleep is when you close your eyes, the lights are out, and your brain is supposedly relaxing. However, sometimes, just because we sleep and then wake up when daylight returns, have we really *'rested?'*

You need adequate rest because it allows your mind and body to relax. Resting helps your body heal and rejuvenate, slowing down aging and repairing cells as well. *Resting is very crucial to our overall wellness.*

The sleep foundation recommends the following to aid in sleeping:

1	*Stick to a sleep schedule of the same bedtime and wake up time, even on the weekends. This helps to regulate your body's clock and could help you fall asleep and stay asleep for the night.*
2	*Practice a relaxing bedtime ritual. A relaxing, routine activity performed right before bedtime and conducted away from bright lights helps separate your sleep time from activities that can cause excitement, stress or anxiety. All of these make it more difficult to fall asleep, get sound and deep sleep, or remain asleep.*
3	*If you have trouble sleeping, avoid naps—especially in the afternoon. Power napping may help you get through the day, but if you find that you cannot fall asleep at bedtime, eliminating even short catnaps may help.*
4	*Exercise daily. Vigorous exercise is best, but even light exercise is better than no activity. Exercise at any time of day as long as it is not at the expense of your sleep.*
5	*Evaluate your room. Design your sleep environment to establish the conditions you need for sleep. Your bedroom should be cool – between 60 and 67 degrees. Your bedroom should also be free from any noise that can disturb your sleep. Finally, your bedroom should be free from any light. Check your room for noises or other distractions. This includes a bed partner's sleep disruptions such as snoring. Consider using blackout curtains, eyeshades, earplugs, 'white noise' machines, humidifiers, fans and other devices.*

6   Sleep on a comfortable mattress and pillow. Make sure your mattress is comfortable and supportive. The one you have been using for years may have exceeded its life expectancy – which is about 9 or 10 years for most good quality mattresses. Have comfortable pillows and make the room attractive and inviting for sleep, but also free of allergens that might affect you. Remove any objects that might cause you to slip or fall if you have to get up in the night.

When we are sleeping, we are increasing our human growth hormones, which is important in slowing the aging process. Sleep also decreases our insulin production. Insulin is more active when we are awake because we are eating and putting sugar and carbs back into our body.

The following diagram illustrates the changes your body goes through in one 24-hour day.

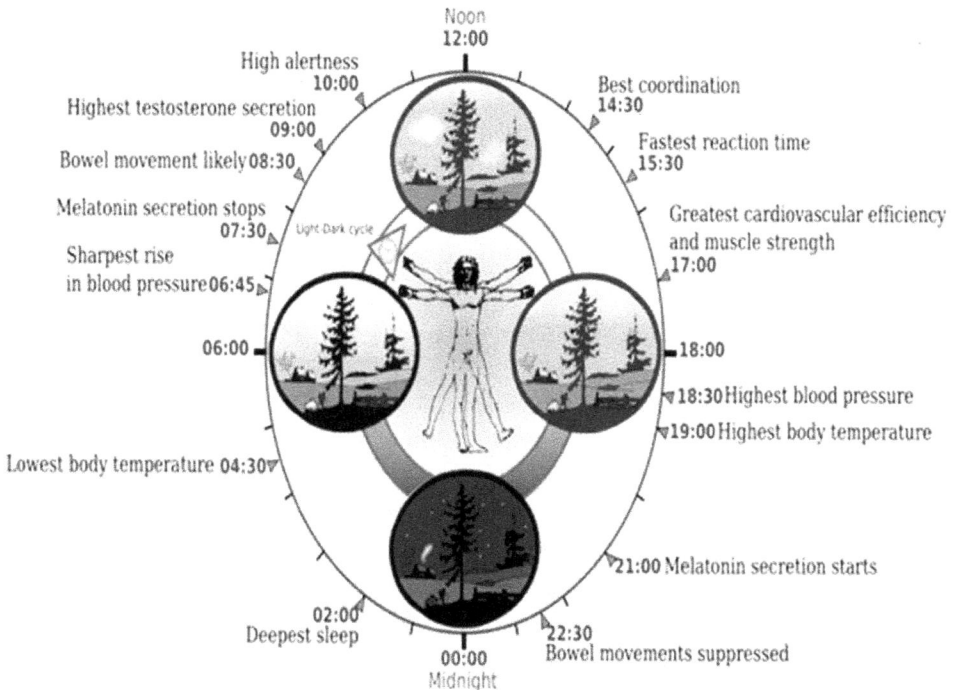

Illustration by: "Biological clock human" by NoNameGYassineMrabetTalk

The Dangers of Not Resting and Sleeping Properly

When you do not get enough sleep, your body cannot rejuvenate as it was intended to do, for proper functioning. When you do not obtain the proper rest, you are endangering yourself and those around you. Some examples of these are below:

Driving	*You are at a greater risk of accidents. According to the National Highway Traffic Safety Administration, fatigue is the cause of 100,000 auto crashes and approximately 1,550 crash related deaths each year in the U.S. alone!*
Poor thinking and decision-making	*Studies show that sleep loss hurts cognitive processes, impairs attention, alertness, concentration, reasoning and problem solving.*
Cooking	*Can lead to burning the food which you're preparing, burning yourself, or causing a fire.*
Workplace	*Depending on the type of work you do, it can indirectly cause detrimental effects to others. For example, if you work in a manufacturing plant and you are not rested, you could miss or skip steps in your normal, regulated routine. Perhaps you may miss assembling a product properly, the item you send out is defective and it causes a problem for the buyer—sometimes a hazardous problem.* *Plus, poor work performance can keep you from getting promoted or recommended for a new job, or may even get you fired, which of course hurts your financial well-being. In another scenario, if your job consists of working with machinery, lifting heavy objects, driving fork-lifts or handling hazardous materials, this can lead to injury or worse—fatalities.*
Health problems	*Sleep deprivation can put you at risk for heart disease, heart attack, heart failure, irregular heartbeat, high blood pressure, stroke, diabetes and more.*

#4 STRESS REDUCTION

This is the fourth and final component of physical wellness. Stress is something we all face, but when it sticks around too long, it can seriously mess with your health.

When we talk about stress, we mean our body's reaction to feeling threatened or under pressure. Our bodies release a hormone called cortisol. Short bursts can help us focus, but when stress hangs around for a long time— that's chronic stress — it starts causing real problems.

How Stress Messes with Your Body	
Chronic stress can mess with your body systems in several ways:	
Heart Health	*It can up your chances of heart disease, high blood pressure, and stroke by making your heart work overtime.*
Immune System	*Stress can knock out your immune system, making you more likely to get sick or stay sick.*
Digestive Issues	*Ever get a stomach ache when you're stressed? It can lead to things like IBS, ulcers, and acid reflux.*
Muscle Tension	*Tension throughout several areas in the body; tension headaches, neck and shoulder tension and all-over body aches.*
Hormonal Havoc	*Stress hormones like cortisol can mess with your metabolism, leading to weight gain and even diabetes.*

Why You Should Care About Stress Reduction	
Taking steps to lower stress isn't just about feeling better right now; it's about keeping your body healthy for the long haul. Here's why it matters:	
Heart Health	*Lowering stress can bring down your blood pressure and heart rate, keeping your heart happier.*

Immune System Boost	*Less stress means a stronger immune system, better able to fight off sickness.*
Happy Gut	*Say goodbye to those stress-related tummy troubles.*
Less Pain	*Relaxing helps ease muscle tension and those pesky headaches.*
Hormone Harmony	*Managing stress helps keep your hormones in balance, which means fewer health issues down the road.*

Kick Stress to the Curb!

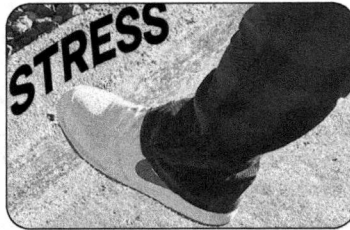

Image Credit: Dr. Wanda Parks

There are tons of ways to lower stress, so you can find one that fits your lifestyle:

Exercise	*Get moving to boost your mood and zap stress.*
Mindfulness and Meditation	*Take time to focus on the now and chill out.*
Deep Breathing	*Slow, deep breaths can calm your mind and body fast. This affects your nervous system.*
Eat Well	*A balanced diet keeps your body strong and your stress levels down. Eating the right foods for your body type is key.*
Sleep Well	*Don't skimp on sleep; it's when your body heals from the day's stress.*

Time Management	*Stay organized to cut down on stress about getting stuff done.*
Socialize	*Hang out with friends and family to feel supported and less stressed.*
Do What You Love	*Hobbies and downtime are great for unwinding and recharging.*

Managing stress isn't just a nice-to-have — it's essential for keeping your body ticking smoothly.

By understanding how stress affects you and using these techniques, you can boost your health and feel better day to day. It's all about setting yourself up for a healthier, happier life.

Let's take some physical action!

PHYSICAL ACTION TASKS

How many times per week do you exercise?

☐ *Never*	☐ *1-2 times*	☐ *3-4 times*	☐ *5-6 times*	☐ *Everyday*

Three times a week is a minimum to get good sleep— at least once per day is optimal.

What does your diet consist of?

1	5
2	6
3	7
4	8

The more fruits and veggies, the better! Try to get the bulk of your protein intake during breakfast and lunch, since protein in the evening can keep you awake. Limit your sugar intake as much as possible. In addition, do not consume caffeine after 1 pm.

What do you do to reduce stress?

1

2

3

Practicing a stress reduction routine daily is beneficial for your well-being.

How many hours of sleep do you get?

☐ *Never*	☐ *1-2 times*	☐ *3-4 times*	☐ *5-6 times*	☐ *Everyday*

The optimal amount can vary from person to person, based on physical activity, wellness, age and so forth. It is best to get to sleep as early as possible and sleep until you wake up naturally, without an alarm clock.

Are you in chronic pain?

☐ *Yes* ☐ *No*

Pain of any kind can make sleep especially difficult. If the pain is treatable with a topical lotion such as Arnica, use it just before bedtime. If the pain is internal, you will want to talk to your doctor about proper pain management.

A note on pain management:

It is surprising how many aches and pains can be alleviated over time by using things like gentle exercise, yoga and stretching.

Yoga especially can be great for things like back, shoulder and leg pain.

Depending on your condition, you might give a gentle yoga program a try by practicing yoga once a day for a month, and seeing if that relieves your pain. You will find plenty of yoga videos on YouTube and in my Holistican membership. Start simple and gentle, and work your way up to more advanced videos and yoga poses over time.

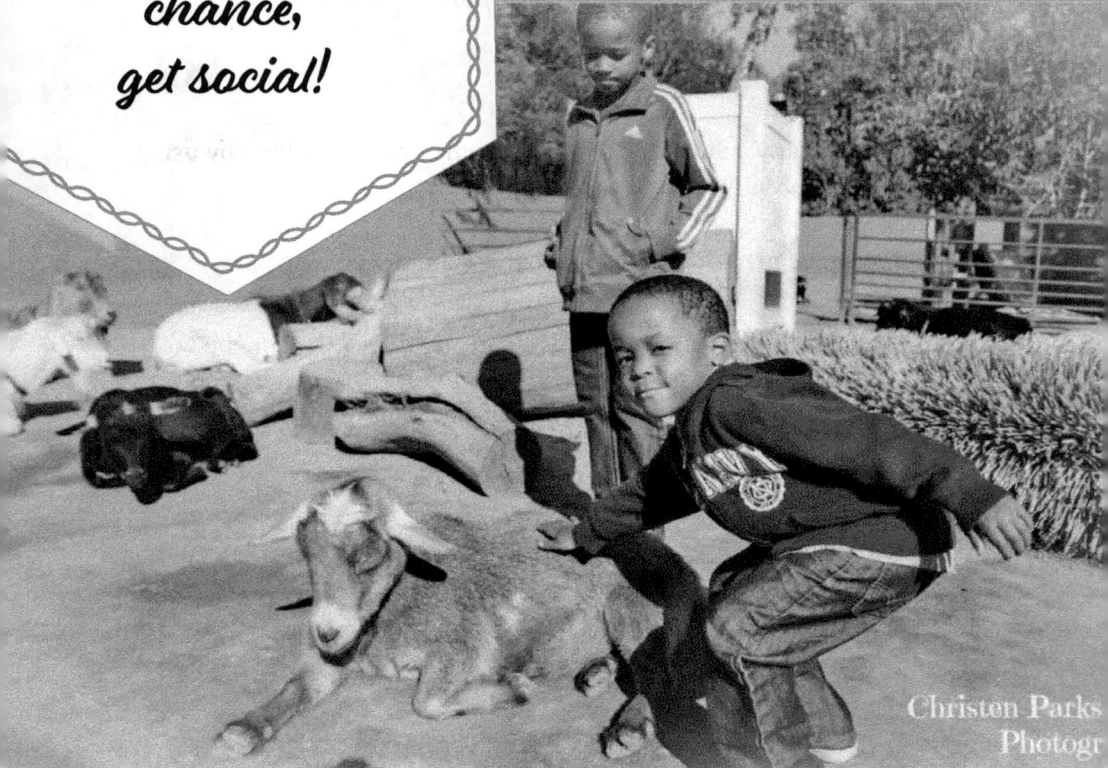

Take a
chance,
get social!

Image Credit:
Christen Parks Photography

3

SOCIAL WELLNESS

Have you lost touch with your high school friends, your zeal for laughter, bantering, and having a good time?

Does your job prevent you from taking that vacation you've dreamed of that would allow you to relax? Have you passed up all invitations to social events except the ones dealing with the children or the corporate office functions? Would you like to do activities that you truly enjoy, but something is stopping you? If that is the case, then your social wellness is affected.

Social wellness is about building deeper bonds with family, coworkers and friends, as well as choosing whom you want in your inner circle. As we all know, when you are being social, you are out mixing and mingling with people. We were not created to be isolated on an island or sitting alone at home all of the time.

> *If you remember, God first created Adam and then the animals. However, God knew that Adam needed a companion, so He created woman. The animals alone were not enough for man. God stated:*
>
> *"It is not good for man to be alone."*
>
> *Genesis 2:18*

Research shows, when people are incarcerated, the isolation has significant negative effects on their mental well-being. As humans, we were made and created to socialize.

A study completed by the University of Chicago, found that at any given time, at least one out of every five persons, or roughly 60 million Americans suffer from loneliness. I know you do not want to be included among those statistics.

Let's examine the word 'sociology.' The root word is '*social.*' You are part of a community; and you are meant to be around people. What happens when you allow yourself to become isolated?

It is unhealthy because you can begin to lose touch with reality. *Your social wellness affects your total wellness.* Isolation becomes detrimental to your health. You may begin to go into a state of depression. You can become phobic, lose touch with reality and experience a mild or severe depression, thereby hurting your overall state of well-being.

When I think of social wellness, I like to compare it to and give you the analogy of someone who has experienced some time in prison. When someone goes to prison, what happens? They are in a small cell for their living quarters, and they only socialize in and with the general populace during the time that is allotted. But when an incident occurs in prison, the offending party may be sent into isolation. Depending upon how long they are reprimanded to be there, they may experience some psychotic mishaps.

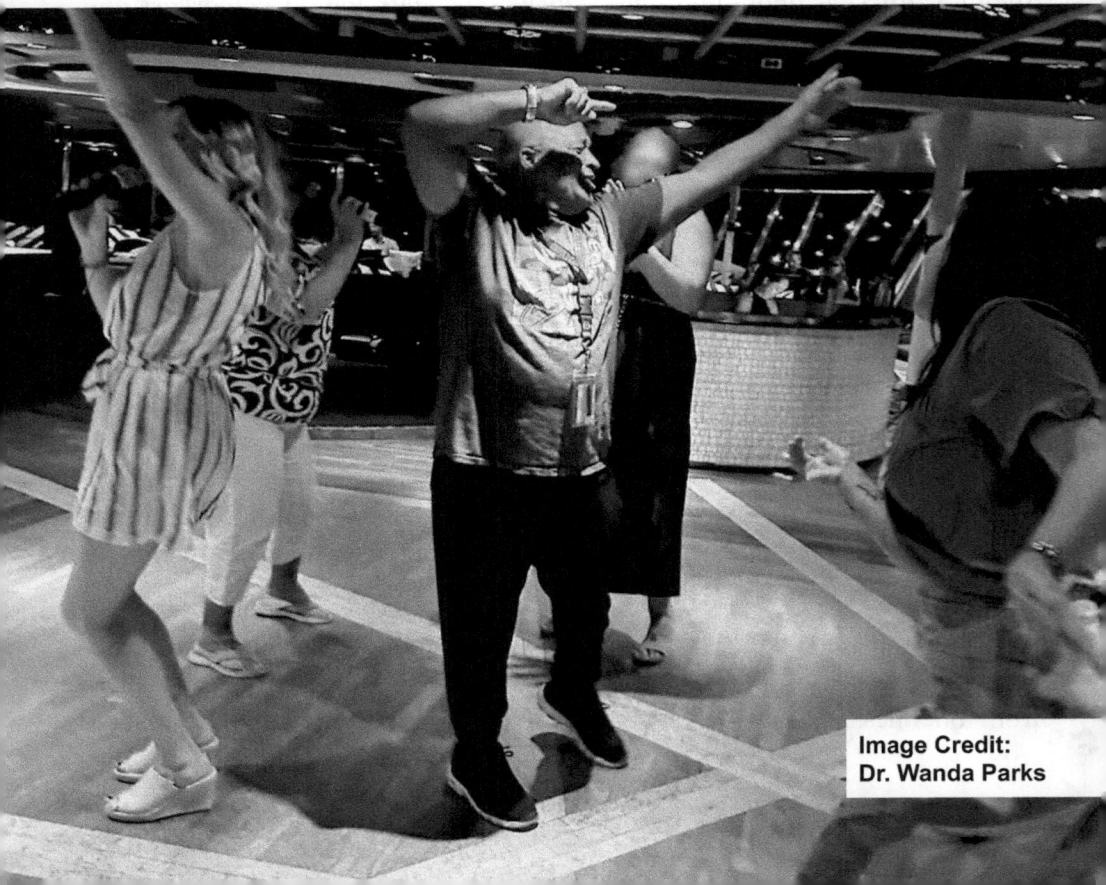

Image Credit:
Dr. Wanda Parks

Some prisoners have psychological issues from being in isolation over extended periods of time. Eventually, when they are released from prison, many are relegated to spend time at what is referred to as a *'halfway house,'* simply because they have to now be resocialized. Another way to look at it is the time spent in isolation *'broke'* them, and now they need to be *'fixed.'*

They have lost the skill set and the mental capability to live within the general, social population as defined by our society. This is a good illustration of exactly how important it is to be among other people, to interact with them, to talk, laugh, share experiences, and connect with others. *It is crucial for your mental well-being.*

BENEFITS OF SOCIAL WELLNESS

The benefits of social wellness allows you to experience life more fully, and enjoy your family and friends. You can actively enhance your mental and physical wellness. A plus is that now you are able to obtain your financial goals and share your life experiences with others.

If you are skeptical of just how important social wellness is, try this experiment: Next time you are feeling a little bit down or depressed, reach out. It does not matter if it is to a friend or a stranger – just have a conversation with someone for at least 5 minutes. Talk about something you enjoy, like the last movie you saw, or about something that interests you— for instance, a social cause.

Then see how you feel compared with how you felt before the interaction. Assuming the person was not a complete downer, I will bet anything you would be feeling less depressed, a bit happier, emotionally lighter and much more optimistic!

Here are steps to enhance your social well-being:

Know your needs:	*We all have unique needs. What someone might deem important may seem irrelevant to you and vice versa. Learn to identify what your needs are so you don't feel the pressure to perform in an environment you don't enjoy or care about.*

Reach out:	*Offering friendship to people is a first step to social wellness. Without this initiative, it would be difficult for you to take advantage of potentially productive relationships. Consider joining groups and clubs that focus on your interests. Explore other avenues that may present certain possibilities for you, such as volunteer work and travel.*
Choose your relationships:	*Some relationships take a toll on people. Sometimes, it could come from experiences with an abusive partner, an overbearing relative or an insincere friend. The problem here is that all of these can cause unnecessary strain on your emotional state and affect your ability to function socially.*
Learn to build and stay in healthy relationships:	*Healthy relationships involve people you care about, who care about you and your well-being. Generally, these are people whom you feel can nurture and support your needs and whose needs you yourself can offer support for. Since there is trust and compassion, you feel safe and satisfied. Two vital ingredients for social wellness.*
Do not feel the pressure to conform:	*This is a rather tricky step because often, conformity is required in the society we live in. However, cooperating with standards and morals doesn't necessarily mean changing yourself and becoming someone you are not. Everyone is different and it is our job to accept that. If you try to conform, you will find that the pressure to change yourself will affect you in many ways, all of them negative.*
Learn to communicate effectively:	*You can only do so much about hiding your feelings and thoughts. Being able to communicate well is a vital component of social wellness because this is generally how you initiate relationships in the first place.*

By understanding how stress affects you and using these techniques, you can boost your health and feel better day to day. It's all about setting yourself up for a healthier, happier life.

SOCIAL ACTION TASKS

Do you take vacations?

☐ *Yes*   ☐ *No*

If not, think about a destination you'd like to visit and consider getting some personalized assistance at: ***successwithwanda.com/glamtravel***

Or do you at least get away now and then on some weekends?

☐ *Yes*   ☐ *No*

If not, you might want to start. If money is tight, consider taking 'stay-cations' where you explore your own community while staying in your home.

Are you involved in social activities and clubs?

☐ *Yes*   ☐ *No*

If not, review the newspaper, or social media for what is happening locally. Join Meetup and search for groups in your area. If you belong to a church, find out what activities they have going on. Join local clubs and if nothing else, start your own groups.

You can start a walking club for your neighborhood, or a social club, or anything you like. Yes, you can even go door-to-door to hand out flyers. It will be a great experience for you, and you will get to meet your neighbors and make new friends.

Enjoy peace
and
tranquility

4

ENVIRONMENTAL WELLNESS

Do you walk into a room and feel disorganized? Is the clutter closing in on you?

If you have trouble finding a space on your desk to set something down, or your kitchen table is chock full of stuff, or you have items crammed into every nook and cranny of your home—it is affecting you in ways you have not even imagined.

Do you walk into a room and smell so many aromas and fragrances, you feel overpowered? Perhaps you feel as if your nasal senses are being attacked. For some of you, your eyes may start to water.

Have you walked down one of the shopping aisles in the store and the smell of the chemicals just overtake you? If you work outside, the pollutants of vehicles passing by can make you cough and make your eyes water. All of this is related to environmental wellness.

Environmental wellness is what surrounds you. It is your environment, which includes your household furnishings, carpets and even your clothes. Chemicals are used in the manufacture of almost everything these days, and breathing these chemicals in, as well as absorbing them through your skin—is taking a toll on you.

Everything around you affects you. It affects your moods, how well you think, your decision-making process, your relationships, and your health.

IS YOUR HOME OR OFFICE CLUTTERED?

Clutter affects your well-being in a variety of ways. It steals your focus by limiting your brain's ability to process information and causing you to

33

feel distracted. It increases stress and overloads your brain. It contributes to procrastination. Clutter costs you time and money. Think of the time you spend searching for things that should be right there at your fingertips. Americans collectively waste 9 million hours per DAY searching for misplaced items. *Nearly one-fourth of us admit to paying late penalties in regards to paying our bills, simply because we could not find the bills prior to their stated 'due dates.'*

We are not done yet… clutter also aggravates your allergies. It is difficult to clean your environment when it is cluttered, hence, germs get to hide in your clutter, triggering allergy and asthma attacks.

Would you believe clutter makes you FAT? Clutter increases your stress hormone, which causes you to gain weight. It also represents bad habits that transfer over to eating patterns as well, leading to the overconsumption of food.

One last note about clutter – it can keep you from living in the present. Clutter is a way of clinging to the past. It represents trapped energy, which is why when you clear clutter, you release negative emotions and generate positive energy while inviting opportunity into your life!

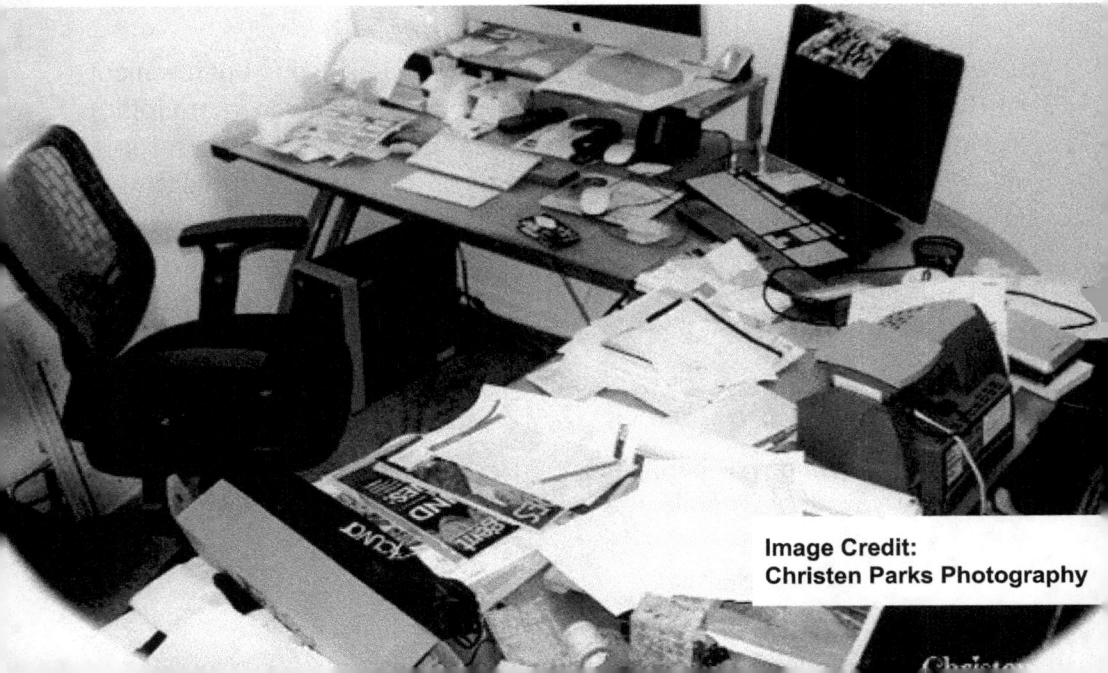

Image Credit:
Christen Parks Photography

CLUTTER ACTION TASKS

This one is super simple—*remove the clutter.*

Okay, I admit that it's easier said than done. Here is how you get started:

Choose the area of your home where you spend the most of your time. This might be your kitchen, your home office, or your bedroom.

Which area of your home will you begin to eliminate clutter?

☐ *Kitchen*   ☐ *Bedroom*   ☐ *Home Office*   ☐ *Other*_____

Start with one area of that room and go through every item, one by one. If you no longer use the item or no longer have any attachment to it, then *thank the item* and *let it go.* Box up all your unwanted and unneeded items and donate them to your favorite thrift store.

Now neatly organize everything that you decide to keep.

Do this in each area of your home, letting go of all the things that no longer serve you. You are going to be pleasantly surprised at how good this process feels and how much better you will feel from here on out when you do this.

INDOOR AIR QUALITY—IT IS WORSE THAN YOU THINK!

We spend more than 90% of our time indoors, yet this is where you will find the worst air quality. In fact, the air inside your home and office is likely 2 to 5 times worse than outside!

Why is indoor air worse than outdoor air? First, windows are generally closed, so we are circulating the same air, dust, skin cells, mites and pollution repeatedly throughout our house.

Second, our homes and offices are filled with chemicals: Laundry soaps, air deodorizers, hair sprays—as well as various types of other spray products such as fragrances, cleaning agents and so forth.

Then there are the chemicals in your furniture and carpet. I will list a few here just to give you an idea of what is lurking in your sofas and tables, but realize this is only the tip of the iceberg:

Volatile organic compounds (VOSs) – *causes eye, nose and throat irritation, headaches, loss of coordination and nausea. May also cause damage to the liver, kidneys and central nervous system.*
Polybrominated diphenyl ethers (PBDEs) – *toxic to both the environment and humans.*
Perfluorinated compounds (PFCs) – *may cause birth defects and cancer.*
Perchloroethylene (PCE) – *can cause dizziness and unconsciousness. Long-term exposure can cause liver and kidney damage, memory loss, confusion and cancer. There is a reason why it has been banned in Canada and Europe.*
Triclosan – *alters hormone regulation.*
Chloride and Ammonia – *long-term exposure can result in lung disease, irritation to skin, eyes, throat and lungs.*

If you are like most people, you are inhaling these chemicals day in and day out, as well as at night when you are sleeping. Your home's air is likely a chemical stew and you do not even realize it.

INDOOR AIR CARE ACTION TASKS

Best defense? First, open windows as often as you can. Second, be very careful when buying new furniture. Do your research. Do not buy carpet without extensively researching exactly what you are bringing into your home.

If you are trapped in an office during the day, open a window if you can. Go outside as much as possible to take your breaks, have lunch and even to make phone calls or catch up on work on your laptop.

Breathing chemicals all day and night will at best make you feel sluggish and tired. It may give you ongoing headaches, as well as other aches and pains. You may have trouble focusing, suffer from foggy thinking, and notice your memory is not what it used to be. You will feel tired. Toxins are one of the prime reasons for fatigue, along with lack of exercise and a poor diet.

Bottom line, spend as much time as you can breathing fresh air and you will feel better. Plus, you will lower your risk of contracting some very nasty, chemically triggered diseases.

Make a list of three actions you can take now for indoor air care:

1.
2.
3.

PERSONAL CARE PRODUCTS—A CHEMICAL STEW!

Did you know there are harmful chemicals in things like hair care products, skin products, make-up, fingernail products, and just about anything you apply to your body?

Did you know that you inhale these chemicals every time you use these products? Worse yet, these chemicals are absorbed through your skin.

And you wonder why you feel so tired and sluggish all of the time!

Here are just a few of the many chemicals to avoid:

Parabens—*found in makeup, moisturizers, shampoos, etc. Interferes with hormone production and may cause breast cancer.*
DEA, cocamide DEA and lauramide DEA, MEA and TEA—*found in creamy and foamy products such as shampoos and moisturizers. Can react to form cancer-causing nitrosamines. Harmful to fish and wildlife.*
Dibutyl Phthalate or DBP—found in nail products and hair sprays. Toxic to reproduction and may interfere with hormone function. Harmful to fish and wildlife.
BHA (butylated hydroxyanisole) and BHT (butylated hydroxytoluene)—*in moisturizers, makeup, etc. Can cause cancer and interfere with hormone function.*
Coal Tar Dyes (P-Phenylenediamine)—*in hair dyes and colors identified as 'C.I.' followed by five digits. Can cause cancer and send heavy metals into the brain. Ouch!*
PEGs (polyethylene glycols, which are petroleum-based compounds)—*found in moisturizers, deodorants, conditioners, etc. Can be contaminated with 1, 4-dioxane, which can cause cancer.*
Formaldehyde-Releasing Preservatives (Dmdm Hydantoin, Diazolidinyl Urea, Imidazolidinyl Urea, Methenamine, or Quaternium-15)—*Used in hair products and causes cancer. By the way, formaldehyde is used to embalm dead bodies. Think about it!*
Synthetic fragrances and Parfum—*would you believe these are even used in products marketed as 'unscented?' That's crazy! The mixture of chemicals in perfumes can trigger allergies and asthma, as well as being linked to cancer and neurotoxicity. They are harmful to fish and wildlife.*

Please don't think the list on the previous page is in any way comprehensive— I've only just begun to scratch the surface of toxic chemicals found in your bathroom.

I have heard some folks say that all these chemicals are no problem – our bodies get rid of them and we are fine. Well, that is not true. Our bodies did not evolve to handle a daily onslaught of hundreds of toxic, man-made chemicals. Therefore, our bodies defend themselves as best they can, by storing many of these chemicals inside fat cells where they remain until something inevitably dislodges them and they run rampant through your body, causing problems. If you were to get tested for all the toxic chemicals known to be in products, you would be shocked at the results!

So what is the solution? Buy organic products that pride themselves on NOT using any of these dangerous chemicals. You can find these products in organic grocery stores and online.

PERSONAL CARE ACTION TASKS

Go through your bathroom and toss out all of the products that you are not sure are safe. Odds are, for most people, this will be most, if not all, of the products in your bathroom right now.

Shop at your local organic grocery store and buy new products that do not contain harmful chemicals.

I know what you are thinking—you are going to be wasting money throwing all this stuff out. However, think of the money, time and your own overall health that you will be saving when you do not get sick, you do not get cancer, you no longer feel tired, and you stop getting headaches. As the saying goes, 'you can pay a little now, or a whole lot later.' Just think of the money you will save by implementing preventative techniques while addressing the root cause of your illness—rather than spending time and money trying to alleviate the pain and other ill effects of not having taken care of your overall health.

While I cannot promise you any of these benefits, I do know for a fact that you are doing the healthiest thing when you eliminate as many toxic chemicals from your life.

Make a list of three actions you can take now for personal care:

1.

2.

3.

CLEANING PRODUCTS

I would be remiss if I did not cover this one as well.

Instead of listing all of the toxic chemicals found in cleaners, let me just share a story with you instead:

At one-time teachers and school janitors were told to use a certain cleaning product in the classroom to kill germs. I am not sure if I'm allowed to use the name without the risk of being sued, but it is a common cleaner that claims to kill germs on contact.

They asked a class of first graders to draw pictures, which they gladly did. The children drew people, pets, houses, and landscapes… all of the things little kids typically draw. Anyone looking at these pictures could tell 9 times out of 10, exactly what the objects in the pictures were supposed to be.

Then they had the students leave the room for a few minutes. While they were gone, they sprayed this particular cleaner in the room. When the children returned, they again asked the kids to draw pictures.

Only this time, the pictures looked like nothing more than random scribbles. Very few objects in the pictures could be deciphered—it was all just random lines and squiggles!

Now if one cleaner used one time can have that much of an effect on children's brains within that short of a time period, do you really think that anyone should be breathing that stuff?

While I wish I could tell you it was only that particular cleaner that's harmful, the fact is nearly every cleaning product out there that is not made from organic ingredients is harmful to breathe, harmful to touch and possibly deadly to ingest!

Why would anyone want these toxins in their home? Because these products happen to have a good commercial on TV? Or perhaps it is simply because it is what you have always used? Because you think that, somehow you are magically protected from these toxins?

Sometimes, like many other habits we possess, the products you use may merely have been handed down from one generation to another. You're aware that your grandparents used them over the years, your parents followed suit and used the same products and now, you continue to use them as well.

While these products may not have appeared to have affected our past generations adversely, we can clearly see the world has changed, and the combination of these deadly toxins are wreaking havoc in many areas of our lives.

Sorry, I'll get off my soapbox now. I am just worried about your health, your family's health, and whether or not you are going to enjoy chemotherapy. (Trust me, you will not!)

Because of my passion for your well-being, remember to check out my recommended reading materials and website links in the back of this book.

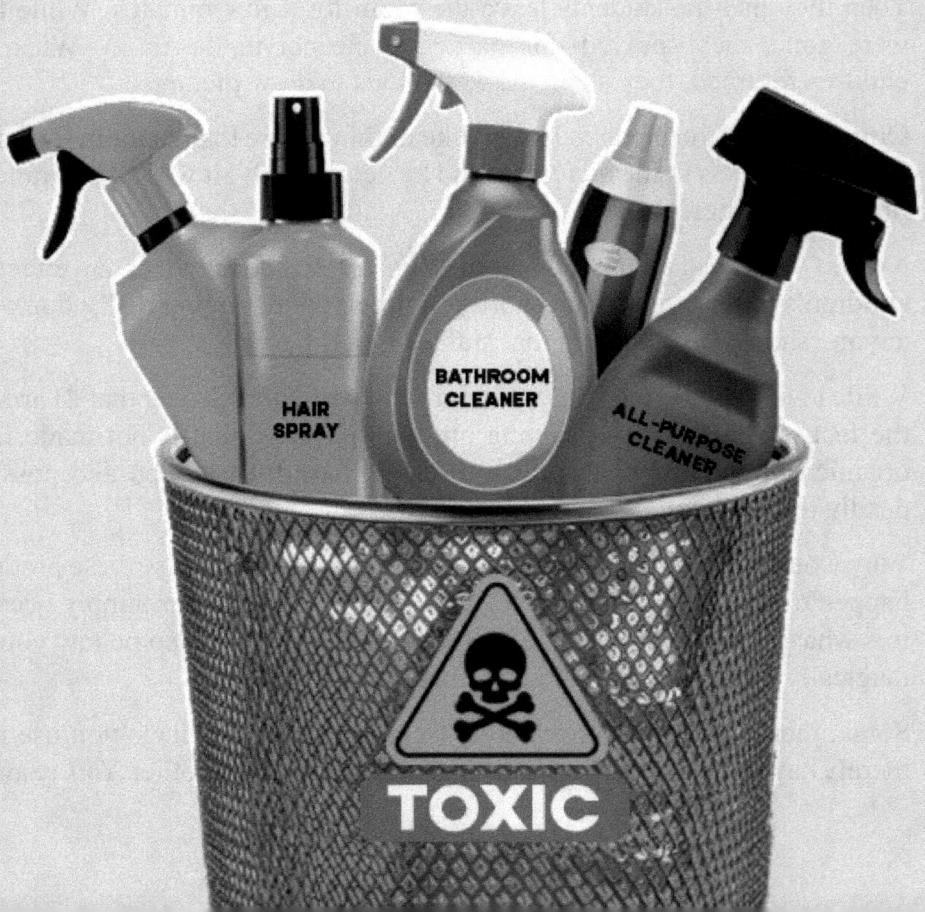

CLEANING PRODUCTS ACTION TASKS

Throw out—and I mean IMMEDIATELY AND WITHOUT HESITATION— throw out every cleaning product in your house that you suspect may be toxic.

Go to your organic grocery store on-line and buy only safe products. Check out the resource page in the back of this book. This is so simple to do, and the health and life you save could be your own.

Yes, I know you think I am over dramatizing. However, after all the research I have done on the topic, I know that these cleaning products are chemical hazards that have no business being anywhere near any living thing. Ever.

List three toxic cleaning products you will remove from your home:

1. _____

2. _____

3. _____

Where do you
find your calm
grounding place?

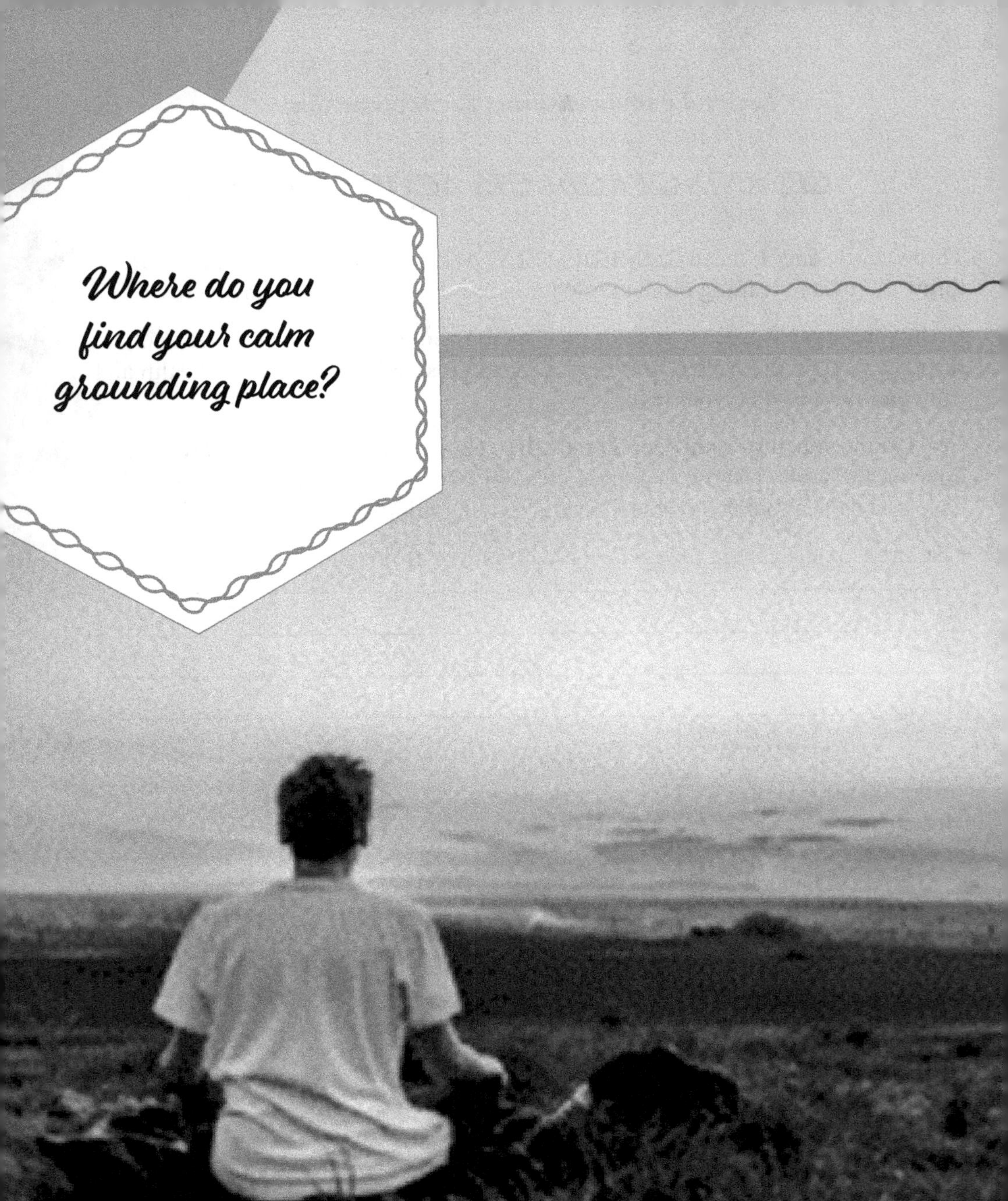

5

SPIRITUAL WELLNESS

Have you ever felt like your life was pure chaos? As if there was nowhere or no one to turn to? Maybe you felt as if you weren't grounded and life was coming at you like a bunch of invisible darts full-speed. You were trying to dodge left and dodge right but to no avail. The darts managed to find you and you have just kept getting hit by them.

Maybe you feel like that right now.

When you feel like that and you cannot figure out where to go or what to do… when you cannot find that calming or grounding moment… this is when your spiritual wellness is where you need to turn.

However, you have to ask yourself, *'Do I have spiritual wellness?'* If so, is your spiritual wellness well and intact?

When you hear the words spiritual wellness, what comes to mind? Many people think spiritual wellness is about religion. There are so many religions out there. Others think of spiritual wellness as a form of meditation. In fact, in some religions, meditation is their spiritual wellness. Offering the Hindu religion as an example, meditation is used for their spiritual wellness. Others chant, like the Buddha's religion.

Spiritual wellness is a personal matter. It involves values and beliefs that give purpose and meaning to our lives. If you think about it, it is better to ponder the meaning of life for ourselves, and to focus on improving ourselves, rather than having closed minds or becoming intolerant of others.

A person who has spiritual wellness will be tolerant of others, regardless of their beliefs and ideas. When you see intolerant people ranting online about "THOSE DAMN PEOPLE," then you know that spiritually, they are not well.

If you have the ability to experience and integrate meaning and purpose into your life, and if you can connect with yourself, and with art, music, literature, and nature, then you have spiritual wellness.

Spiritual wellness for me is the place you go for hope and answers, to help you when you are struggling through life. It is the place where you feel calm and centered. Think of your inner self, of being healed within, of feeling at one with everyone around you, of being a part of something vastly greater than yourself. That, to me, is spiritual wellness. I know that some often interchange spirituality and religion as one in the same. While researching, I came across two views—one of religion and one of spirituality.

Émile Durkheim's explains religion:

'A religion is a unified system of beliefs and practices relative to sacred things, that is to say, things set apart and forbidden -- beliefs and practices which unite into one single moral community called a Church, all those who adhere to them.'

While sociologist Flora Timmins et al. explains that spirituality:

'Arises from personal beliefs, which may result from an individual's religious beliefs, background, or childhood.'

In today's society, we are adopting some of these religious traditions into daily practice in making us well. This plays a factor in your overall wellness because your spiritual wellness is tapping into your inner self. It is the calm within. Meditation helps calm you.

It centers you and reduces your heart rate, helps with your blood pressure, and helps with weight loss. It helps in decreasing your stress levels and your cortisol levels—things that can affect your health. With our crazy day-to-day living and the hustle and bustle, we forget to take time to find the calm and the grounding we need. Some may turn to meditation. There are different types of meditation that people can do to help with their well-being such as focus meditation, mindful meditation or transcendental meditation, and others.

You can incorporate your spiritual wellness practice in the morning, in the afternoon, or in the evening. Your spiritual wellness is an important factor that some have failed to recognize and implement in their well-being.

We only get one body, and the one body that we have is our temple. As Christians, we are taught that our body is our temple, and we need to keep it holy and clean and revere it. Let's face it; we put so many things in our bodies that are not healthy for us. We are not doing what we are instructed to do to keep this temple holy, or clean. We have to do better. Well, at least I know I will be more cognizant and work towards keeping my temple in tip-top shape.

> *Do you not know that you are a temple of God and that the Spirit of God dwells in you? If any man destroys the temple of God, God will destroy him, for the temple of God is holy, and that is what you are.*
>
> *1 Corinthians 3:16-17*

Our bodies have so many chemicals from our environment, as well as all of the pollutants that affect our bodies on a daily basis. We forget that we need to take care of our bodies on a regular basis.

BENEFITS OF SPIRITUAL WELLNESS

Here are some ways to find spiritual health:

Be still and quiet
Be open to others and new possibilities
Look for the deeper meanings in life
Write down your thoughts and emotions to help you clarify what is happening and to focus on what is important
Practice being non-judgmental and having an open mind
Be receptive to pain or times of sorrow (this too, shall pass)
Practice forgiveness. Not for the other person so much, but also for yourself and your well-being
Pray, meditate, or worship as you see fit
Live joyfully

Smile, even when you don't feel like it, as this will cause you to feel more positive
Try yoga or Tai Chi
Live in the present moment, and not in the future or past
Love yourself so that you may love others
Travel – it can do wonders for your mind while allowing you to de-stress, reflect and rest
Watch uplifting movies, read uplifting books and articles
Practice positive thinking – when a negative thought intrudes, replace it with a positive thought
Listen to your inner voice
Talk to God, the universe, or even yourself (It's highly therapeutic!)
Be grateful and do not take anything for granted
Laugh. Laugh out loud a lot, sing, and dance as if no one is watching

SPIRITUAL ACTION TASKS

What do you do to relieve stress?

_____

_____

_____

_____

If the answer is 'nothing,' then maybe it is time you took up some new hobbies such as walking in nature, meditation, or yoga.

How do you define spiritual wellness?

_____

_____

_____

_____

What is important to you?

_____

_____

_____

_____

Spiritual wellness is different for everyone, so I do not have a pat answer for you. Rather, I would suggest you look within and find out what makes you spiritually happy and at peace with the world and with yourself.

What do you do, or practice, to help in finding your center?

_____

_____

_____

_____

_____

☐ *Yes*   ☐ *No*   Do you feel grounded?

☐ *Yes*   ☐ *No*   Do you have a place to turn to when life is closing in?

Whatever the case may be for you personally, truly explore the many avenues and opportunities available for you to begin this important journey of discovering what spiritual wellness means for you.

For some, it is hiking in nature. For others, it is visiting their church. Yet for others, it could be going to a special place in your mind and heart.

The first step in
Financial
Wellness
is starting

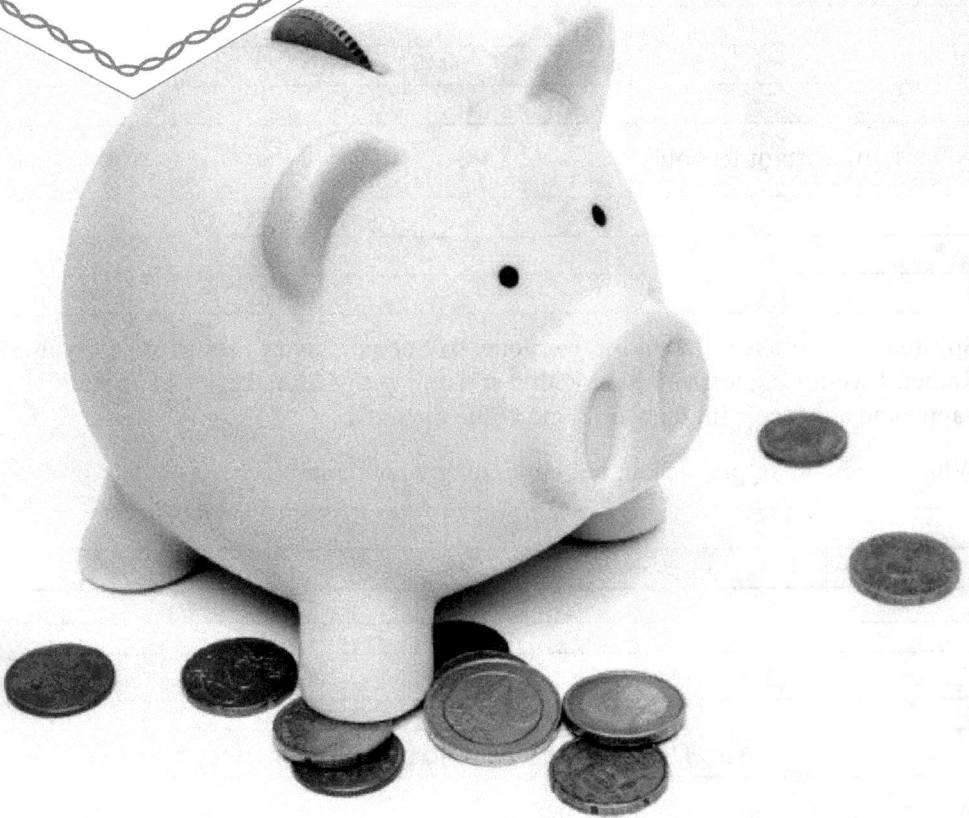

6

FINANCIAL WELLNESS

Financial wellness should be very important to you because you must have ample finances to survive. The world runs on a financial economy.

If you do not have enough money to maintain your lifestyle, your finances are not well, and you are not going to be able to complete some of the other parts of your wellness plan. If you are in a lot of debt, chances are, you are going to be stressed and depressed and you are not going to want to get out and do anything. This is why you have to have financial wellness, as it plays an important part in your overall well-being.

Take a look at your budget and review your spending habits. Prepare to get your financial wellness intact. Do not live above your means. Dave Ramsey speaks about being financially well. His Financial Peace University is a great program to assist you in getting your financial wellness intact.

Start your emergency fund. Take those baby steps that are needed for you to pay down and eventually pay off, your outstanding debt. Once you do that, you are now able to delve into your physical wellness, spiritual wellness, environmental wellness, mental wellness, and social wellness. When you have financial wellness, you are able to do the things that you long to do without stressing yourself out. When your financial wellness is in balance and intact, your other wellness components have the capacity to also be good. When you are not financially well, it can cause undue strain on your relationships and impact your children. At times, you do not eat well because you cannot afford the healthier food options available in the marketplace.

Worse yet, you tend to make poor choices because you are upset about not being financially well. You do not travel where you want to go, simply because you do not have the finances to do so. It is a cascading effect that affects you and your entire family when you do not have your financial wellness intact.

Determine the things you truly need, as well as those items you do not need, and those things that you can do without. Learn how to manage your finances better for you and your family. Create the kind of financial well-being that allows you to take those family vacations and those romantic evenings with your loved one. You are then able to do the things that you want to do, travel to the places that you want to travel to, and begin to enjoy the type of entertainment that suits you!

For some, it's as simple as increasing your income while not increasing your spending. You can use the extra money you earn to invest in your financial future, purchase a home, and pay off debt... anything that will make you more financially secure and 'well.'

Here is a brief list of ways you can earn more money, many of which you can implement this month:

Ask for a raise
Secure a new job that pays better
Obtain a part-time job, such as doing customer service by phone from your home
Become a virtual assistant
Start a blog and promote affiliate products
Run errands or do odd jobs for people
Sell the things you no longer need on Craigslist or eBay
Review Craigslist for good deals, then resell those items for more money
Become a pet sitter
Do freelance writing
Become a driver for Uber, Lyft, or SideCar
Rent out your car on Turo, JustShareIt, or GetAround
Rent out your house on Airbnb
Reduce your expenses
Become an online tutor
Sell information products online

Start an online membership site
Teach online courses
Do odd jobs posted on Craigslist
Resell items from thrift stores
Design and build websites
Turn your commute or road trip into money by delivering items through Roadie
Sell your old books using BookScouter to find which online buy-back site will pay the most

In addition, here are some quick financial tips to get you on the right path:

Pay off higher interest rate loans first
Track your net worth. Anything you track grows
Make a calendar or reminders to tell you when to pay quarterly bills, when to pull your credit reports, and so forth
If you have not started planning for retirement, start today, regardless of how old or young you may be
Set a budget and stick to it. Period
Pay yourself first. Every time you are paid, set aside 10% for yourself
If you are a tither, then also tithe your 10%
Use only cash. When we pull out the plastic, it does not seem real. However, when we hand the cashier real money, we quickly realize what we are spending. This small change can make a big difference in how much you spend!
Check on your finances daily. Spending just a few minutes each day tracking your financial transactions, keeps your money on your mind. You will begin to spend less and save more when you do this
Make a financial vision board. This will help you to stay on track immensely

Set financial goals using numbers AND dates. Make big goals and break them down into bite-sized goals
Before making a purchase, ask yourself if you really want or need the item. If you are not sure, put it back. If you really want it, you can go back and get it later. However, 9 times out of 10 you will not
Banish all toxic money thoughts, such as, 'I'll never get this paid off.'
Exercise. Crazy as it sounds, the better shape you are in, the more money you will tend to make because you are able to be more productive and think better
Appreciate what you have now, versus what you might buy in the future
Get a money buddy and keep each other accountable
Negotiate a raise as well as better benefits. Emphasize the value you bring to the company
Do you have mountains of debt? Pay off the smaller ones first – that will give you the confidence to pay off the larger ones as well
Do not cosign for anyone. If the person misses payments, it will destroy your credit and your relationship with that person
Do not buy a new car when your current car is paid off and still getting you around. No, you do not need to keep up with the neighbors, so just don't. Let them make car payments, not you
If you are buying a car, buy a used one. New cars depreciate on average 19% in the first year. It's simply not worth it
Quality is more important than trendiness. Buying something that will last for the long haul will also save you money and prevent you from having to waste time and money buying another one later
Shop alone. Have you ever had a friend say, "That is so cute, you should buy it?" Socialize in other ways and you will not buy stuff you will regret

Start saving now. Today. Right now. This minute!

FINANCIAL ACTION TASKS

☐ *Yes*   ☐ *No*   Are you working full or part-time?

☐ *Yes*   ☐ *No*   Do you want to work more hours?

☐ *Yes*   ☐ *No*   Would you like to ask for a raise?

☐ *Yes*   ☐ *No*   Are you looking to work a second job or start a business?

The possibilities are nearly endless, and the key is to decide and then take action.

☐ *Yes*   ☐ *No*   Do you have credit cards?

Get out all of your credit card statements and see how much you owe. Then make a plan to pay it all off as soon as possible.

☐ *Yes*   ☐ *No*   Are you saving and investing?

If not, the time to start is today!

☐ *Yes*   ☐ *No*   Does thinking of money freak you out?

If you look away when walking by the financial section in the bookstore, you probably have money issues. *It is time to start reading about how money works and getting used to the idea of making more money, investing that money, and making it grow.*

☐ *Yes*   ☐ *No*   Did your parents tell you that money is the root of all evil?

Read some financial prosperity books and turn your money attitude around. You can do it. It will just take time, and it is well worth it. After all, you do not want to retire financially broke, nor do you want to remain in a financial situation whereby one circumstance—one emergency or one unexpected 'life happening' event, could send you into a financial tailspin, or ruin all that you've worked so hard towards.

Now that you have the foundation it's time for...

YOUR BETTER NEXT STEP

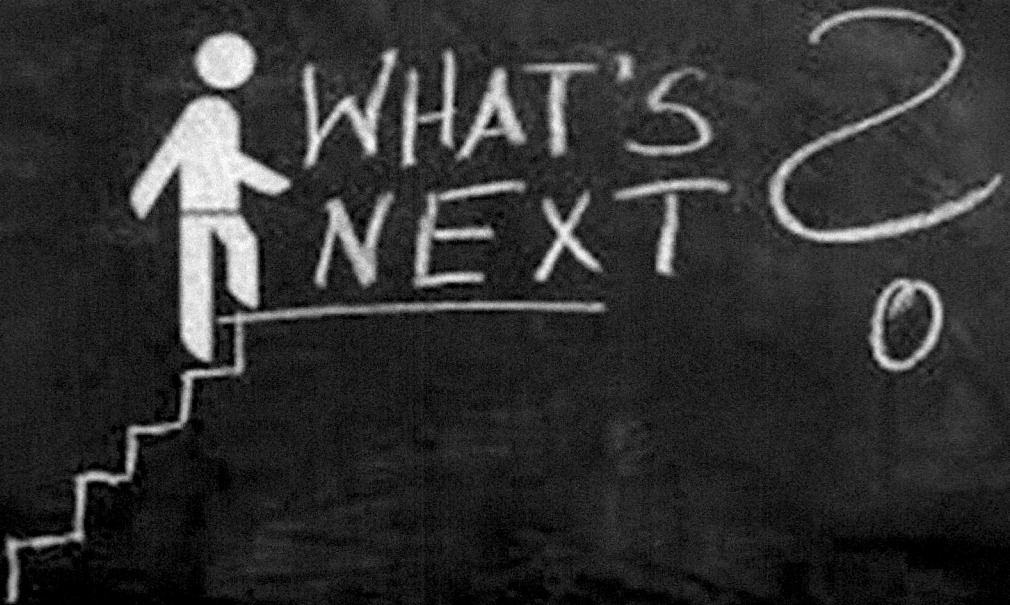

Your Better Next Step

INTRODUCTION

Now that you have gone through the foundational steps and completed your action tasks, you may be asking what is my better next step? Well, many believe that medication is the next step to completing their wellness goal, but I am here to tell you that your better next step is an integrated one. We have to shift the way we look at the body, we have to know it is an individual machine that is wonderfully made by our God. You are not a robot.

> *In Psalm 139, David's prayer to God says,*
> *"I am fearfully and wonderfully made."*
>
> *This speaks of the care and attention with which God has made us. By now, God has made billions of human beings, but we're not mass-produced. We're not churned out in a mechanistic way.*
>
> *~www.crossway.org~*

We need to ensure that all the spark plugs (body systems)—nervous system, cardiovascular system, immune system, musculoskeletal system, integumentary system, digestive system, urinary system, and endocrine system — are firing correctly. So, before diving deeper into this, I want to share my journey and how I developed the 5R method, where I use a functional, holistic, and integrative approach to improve my health using functional screenings.

Now a 24-year veteran, I was an air force nurse, a flight nurse to be specific, and this is when I was placed on my first forever medication when I woke up with a frozen index finger. I had to wait an entire weekend to be seen at the flight clinic. Over the course of time walking became excruciating and I was unable to walk or barely stand. I hid this very well but those close to me could see it on my face. This led to an increase in anxiety, depression and fear. Fear of being discharged from the military. I could not believe this was happening to me.

This was one of my worst nightmares…I wanted to complete my career. I began the journey to improve my health and well-being. After being placed on a chemotherapy drug, which then went into weekly injections. This cascade of events was so crazy to me. My head was spinning in disbelief. I was also placed on depression and anxiety medication as well as medication to counteract the side effects of those medications. I was on a crazy roller coaster and I don't like roller coasters, so I wanted off.

I knew I had to make a decision to do something different without being placed on any additional medication. I made a decision and took charge of my health and well-being and began to do the work.

See, most people believe that once they are diagnosed with a disease, they are trapped and must stay on the hamster wheel of trial and error.

However, there are several things that have to be done, and it is a process. There is no magic bullet or pill; if so, then the world would not be sick… wouldn't you agree? However, with evolving technology and the post-industrial revolution, we have become sicker instead of healthier, and everyone is looking for that magic bullet.

I began tapping into aromatherapy, biofeedback, meditation, and delving into looking at health from a different perspective. I invested nearly $90K in finding a method to improve my health. Most people look at improving their health as a cost, but consider this: you will pay for care either way… to treat your illness or prevent it. You have to make a decision.

So, which would you choose? I like to call this the now or later concept. Think of it, if you pay for prevention now you can continue to do the things you want to do with your loved ones and friends without someone having to wipe your behind [booty], help you get dressed, or pay later when you will need someone to wipe your behind, and may have to provide so much more care to you because you can't walk, are inflamed and in constant pain with a plethora of other ailments. You will miss out on so many activities with the people you love. Ask yourself…

Are you playing checkers or chess with your health? Playing checkers is easy and doesn't take a lot of work. But playing chess is a strategic game and it's not as quick as many play the game over days.

Now let me be clear, I don't have a miracle solution, but I can offer you insight into how your remarkably designed system functions and provides strategies to reignite your inner spark and restore your vitality.

Many may have worked with someone and seen some results only to revert to where they were or hit what I call a flat spot. Also, some may not have done anything because they don't know where to start.

I find having this three-leg approach—the right program, support, and accountability invaluable to my clients and any program:

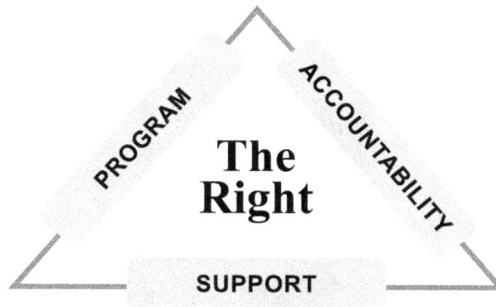

Figure 7-1: Three-leg approach

If one of these components is missing, then the results will be tilted. Although we find a program or a solution we think will fix us, only to find one of the legs is missing.

So, you may ask, what is MY better next step?

I'm here to tell you...

FUNCTIONAL LAB SCREENINGS

The public is crying out for help. Many are tired of all the medications they have been placed on and not getting results. You may feel like you're just treating or suppressing the symptoms that are the cause of your health problems. I'm not against medication; however, we must first consider lifestyle and this should be our first step to improving our wellbeing and taking care of our temple.

As an FDN practitioner, there are three components to providing Functional lab screenings. Which are broken down into three components: **F**unctional, **D**iagnostic, and **N**utrition. These are the foundational components I utilize with clients. Let's take a closer look at what each of these terms mean:

Functional	Diagnostic	Nutrition
This term signifies an approach that works with and respects the innate intelligence of the body. It emphasizes understanding how the body truly operates, its functions, and its natural inclination toward achieving equilibrium and balance (homeostasis).	*This term refers to a process that is diagnostic in nature, rather than a medical diagnosis. Combined with a functional approach, it aims to uncover health revitalization opportunities by identifying and addressing factors that may hinder the body's natural healing response and recovery process.*	*Nutrition involves nurturing and feeding the body's cells, tissues, organs, and systems. It is about providing all the essential elements that the body, both genetically and spiritually needs to thrive and maintain optimal health. We must fuel every cell with the right food for our metabolic type.*

Why Do You Need Functional Screenings?

It depends, are you ready to find health revitalization opportunities? Then your answer should be yes. If you want to stay on the same trajectory and continue to play checkers then the answer is no.

Functional lab screenings allow the practitioner to identify health revitalization opportunities and resolve the most common health complaints at the causal level. Anyone can run labs, but without a complete understanding, most providers just end up treating the test results, the paper instead of the person. Functional screening bridges the gap between medical care and self-care.

Struggles/Challenges

Why don't we opt-in to the true self-care models? Many face challenges or struggles when it comes to improving their health and well-being because of several factors, this can be one by itself or a combination of the following: finances, fear, commitment, and accountability.

Finances	*Most people struggle with looking at improving their health because they look at it as a cost rather than an investment. Also, because many holistic practitioners do not take insurance this leads to many people continuing to suffer or struggle to feel better without using a more alternative approach. Due to this fact, many insurance companies do not favor this approach. However, some people may use their FSA/HSA card as long as it has the capability of being used and processed as a credit card.*
Fear	*Having fear is due to you may be stepping into an unknown territory of holistic approach to wellness and being that many turn to 'uncle' Google who has displayed many negative views on the holistic approach that people believe. Also, there is a fear of trusting someone to help them.*
Commitment	*Many are not truly committed to the process. Once things get a bit tough, many stop. One of the legs is missing or there are some personal obstacles that may impede one's commitment.*
Accountability	*When you have accountability, you have a higher chance of reaching your wellness goal. This is because we never want to let someone down or disappoint them. This can also be an extrinsic motivating factor.*

If you can get past these struggles, you will be on your way to building optimal health and creating your wellness lifestyle. If you have any of the above struggles/challenges then you may need support to help you reach your wellness goals.

The Solution

As you heard my story at the beginning of this chapter, you have to know what you are treating rather than throwing spaghetti at the wall and hoping it sticks. You have to be ready to play chess and give up playing checkers.

I have created the '5Rs to Holistic Wellness' that addresses the problem, not just the symptoms. This 5-phase process includes recognize, roadmap, roll out, refinement, and retention. We have to look beneath the iceberg, as that is where the fire is brewing. The symptoms you are experiencing are a result of the problem, just letting you know that a spark plug is in need of some attention.

To start this process, you have to first **recognize** that there is a problem. Secondly, you have to have a **roadmap** to show you where to go. Third, you will **roll it out** and start the drive. As you go along, there will be some **refinement** as things improve, which is the fourth step. Lastly, you must **retain** what you have done.

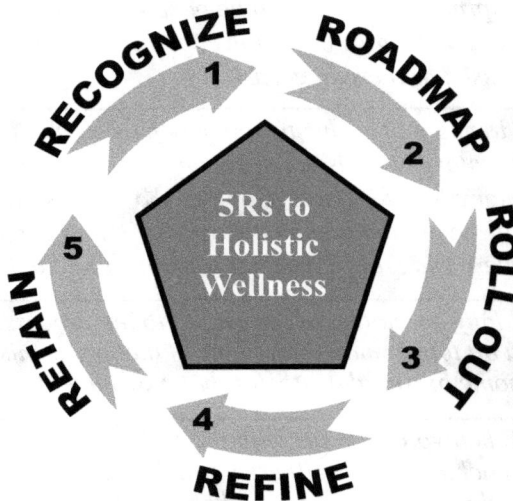

Figure 7-2: The 5R Method℠ to Holistic Wellness

Find someone you are comfortable with to help you on the path to success utilizing functional labs in your well-being and health. Just be aware their approach may be different.

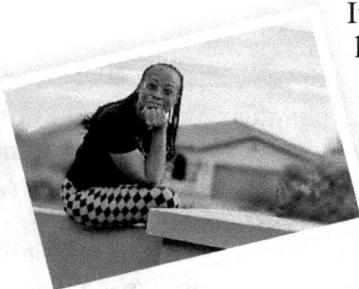

If you are serious about your health and want to keep the body functioning at its optimal level then this is the way to go. Stop sitting on the wall! Move toward Your Better Next Step and order your Wellness Audit today.

Image credit: Dr. Wanda Parks

YOUR BETTER NEXT STEP ACTION TASKS

What does the word HOLISTIC mean to you?

_____

_____

_____

_____

_____

☐ *Yes*　　　☐ *No*　Have you ever worked with a functional wellness/health
coach/practitioner?

_____

If yes, what were the results? If no, why not? _____

_____

_____

_____

What is your biggest health complaint/frustration you want resolved? _____

_____

_____

_____

Select the struggles/challenges you are facing [select all that apply]
☐ Finance
☐ Fear
☐ Commitment
☐ Accountability

On a scale of 1-10, how ready are you to move forward with your better next step?

☐ 1-4	☐ 5-6	☐ 7-10
Not at all, I like where I am	*I am straddling this fence*	*I am so ready no matter what the investment*

If you're a 5 or above have you taken the '*Revitalized*　☐ *Yes*　　☐ *No*
Your Health Wellness Audit' from Dr. Wanda?

If *No*, having a Wellness Audit may help you gain
clarity on your wellness concerns.

ORDER TODAY!
https://solo.to/drwanda

CONCLUSION

Now that you have read and completed this book, true wellness is probably more than you may have ever imagined. If even just one of these six spectrums is out of sync, it can take a toll on your overall lifestyle and well-being.

In order for you to accomplish and live the wellness lifestyle, you must give each of the action steps your best shot. When you do, you'll find all areas of your life improving, especially your health.

The one thing that I know is that the first area—mental wellness, and the last—financial wellness, are a must, in order to accomplish the remaining areas I've discussed in-between these two, in relation to your overall health and wellness.

No matter what ailments you encounter, keeping your mental wellness intact allows you to enjoy a greater quality of life. Personally, I do not want to be a burden on my family as I age gracefully, and I know that an ounce of prevention is worth a ton of cure.

Please do not take these suggestions lightly. You picked up this book because you wanted to change something in your lifestyle and well-being.

Honestly, results won't happen overnight. You have to be consistent and nurture each area. I continually work on every area of my wellness to stay balanced in mind, body, and spirit—and I know you can do the same. Connect with me and I can further assist you.

If you are ready to embark on a true wellness journey and want to have personal access to me for coaching, grab either one or both of these programs: *The 90-day Body Awareness Gut Detox,* or *The Gut Buster Plan.* You can also become a part of my Facebook group: "Holistic Healing; Conquering Metabolic & Autoimmune Conditions."

ADDITIONAL AUTHOR INFORMATION

In addition to being a successful author, speaker, and wellness coach, Wanda Parks' life journey and experiences include having achieved:

PhD	*(Doctor of Philosophy)*
I-MD	*(Doctorate in Integrative Medicine)*
MA	*(Master of Arts in Military Operations)*
MA	*(Master of Arts in Human Resource Management)*
BS	*(Bachelor of Science Holistic Health)*
BSN	*(Bachelor of Science in Nursing)*
RN	*(Registered Nurse)*

Wanda is a member of the following organizations:

Alliance of International Aromatherapists (AIA)
Academy Medical-Surgical Nurses (AMSN)

Combining her love for luxury travel and her passion for assisting others to do so, Wanda obtained the following achievements:

TRAVEL CREDENTIALS
Cruise Line International Association (CLIA)
Travel Tourism Diploma
Travel Agency Proficiency (TAP)
Travel Institute Member
MSC Cruise Specialist
Well-being Travel Specialist
Luxury Travel Specialist
Master Cruise Counselor (MCC)

WANDA'S RECOMMENDATIONS

It is my hope you were able to enjoy this book and that you have been inspired to empower change in your life. I would like to give you some additional resources that I believe will add to and enhance your healthy lifestyle.

Mindset and Meditation- A Journaling Experience
Red Smoothie Detox Recipes
100 Healthy Snacks—No baking required!
Moms Wanting Financial Wellness
Wellness Shopping Club

FOR MORE INFO VISIT
https://solo.to/drwanda

Pick up your FREE Weight-loss Guide

DOWNLOAD GUIDE
https://solo.to/drwanda

Contact Dr. Wanda

SEND AN E-MAIL
info@successwithwanda.com

Free Holistic Healing Facebook community

JOIN THE FREE COMMUNITY
https://solo.to/drwanda

Choose how you wish to connect with Dr. Wanda!
Instagram / TikTok / YouTube

FOLLOW WANDA ON SOCIAL
https://solo.to/drwanda

INTENTIONALLY LEFT BLANK